WHAT
YOU
REALLY
REALLY
WANT

THE SMART GIRL'S

SHAME-FREE GUIDE

TO SEX AND SAFETY

BY JACLYN FRIEDMAN

SEAL PRESS

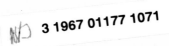

What You Really Really Want
The Smart Girl's Shame-Free Guide to Sex and Safety

Published by
Seal Press
A Member of the Perseus Books Group
1700 Fourth Street
Berkeley, California

Library of Congress Cataloging-in-Publication Data

Friedman, Jaclyn.
  What you really really want : the smart girl's shame-free guide to sex and safety / by Jaclyn Friedman.
    p. cm.
  Includes bibliographical references and index.
  ISBN 978-1-58005-344-0 (alk. paper)
  1. Sexual ethics for women. 2. Women--Sexual behavior. 3. Sex. 4. Sexual health. 5. Sex instruction for women. I. Title.
  HQ46.F77 2011
  176'.4082--dc23

                                    2011030552

9 8 7 6 5 4 3 2 1

Cover design by BriarMade
Interior design by www.meganjonesdesign.com
Printed in the United States of America
Distributed by Publishers Group West

PRAISE FOR WHAT YOU REALLY REALLY WANT

"Jaclyn Friedman is my new hero. As someone who teaches under-graduates, what I really really want is to hand out complimentary copies of this book to all my women students. But I'll settle for dog-eared copies in every college and university Women's, Gender, and Sexuality Resource Center."

—Lyn Mikel Brown, Ed.D., cofounder of SPARK, professor of education and Women's, Gender, and Sexuality Studies, Colby College

"Friedman's new guide—detailed, intelligent, and fun as hell to read—is a sorely needed addition to any bookshelf. Think of it as the anti-Cosmopolitan: A 21st-century primer on fearlessly discovering and owning your sexuality while staying true to yourself without cutesy gimmicks, absurd tips, and patronizing assumptions.

—Anna Holmes, founding editor, Jezebel.com

"In a better world, your sexuality would start as a blank canvas where only you painted the picture . . . and the world in which that painting existed would be free of art critics. Unfortunately, we don't live in that world. The good news is that Friedman has provided a powerful panacea to that world, one that can help you become the master artist of a healthy sex life that's of your own design."

—Heather Corinna, executive director, Scarleteen, and author of S.E.X.

"Friedman challenges readers to rethink how they make sense of their bodies, sexuality, and gender, all the while offering an honest take on the risks involved, like sexual assault and STIs. By teaching girls how to become more attuned with their own bodies and sexualities, Friedman doesn't just give readers the tools to say no to social expectations and gender roles, she teaches them how to say yes to their desires—the very definition of empowerment!"

—Lena Chen, blogger, SexAndTheIvy.com

For K, C, E, and S

TABLE OF CONTENTS

INTRODUCTION
IS THIS BOOK FOR ME? | 1

CHAPTER 1
YOU CAN'T GET WHAT YOU WANT
TILL YOU KNOW WHAT YOU WANT | 13

CHAPTER 2
BAD THINGS COME IN THREES: SHAME, BLAME, AND FEAR | 45

CHAPTER 3
I'M OKAY, YOU'RE OKAY | 71

CHAPTER 4
A WOMAN'S INTUITION | 99

CHAPTER 5
WHAT'S LOVE GOT TO DO WITH IT? | 129

CHAPTER 6
FREAKS AND GEEKS | 157

CHAPTER 7
LET'S TALK ABOUT SEX, BABY | 187

CHAPTER 8
IT'S COMPLICATED | 221

CHAPTER 9
DO UNTO OTHERS | 253

CHAPTER 10
FRIENDS AND FAMILY | 281

CHAPTER 11
TO INFINITY AND BEYOND | 311

NOTES | 335

IS THIS BOOK FOR ME?

O KAY. SO YOU'RE INTRIGUED. MAYBE A LITTLE SUSPICIOUS. Something about this book made you want to pick it up and open it, but hey—that's probably true of a lot of books. I get it.

So let's cut to the chase. Answer the ten questions below to find out if this book is for you. For each question, pick an answer that's closest to what's true for you. If a particular question doesn't relate to your present life, then imagine how you might answer it if it did. Be honest—no one's looking!

1. You're single and you're going to a party where there may be people you'd be attracted to. Do you dress sexy?

   a. *You know it!*
   b. *If I'm feeling brave.*
   c. *It depends on what you mean by sexy.*
   d. *Probably not. I'd feel too foolish or shy.*
   e. *No way. I don't want to give anyone the wrong impression.*

2. Telling someone what you want to do with them (or what you want them to do with you) sexually is:

   a. *Hot.*
   b. *Scary.*
   c. *A total buzzkill.*
   d. *Something I wish I could do.*
   e. *My favorite way to spend an evening.*

3. You do things sexually that feel okay at the time, but you feel bad about it afterward.

   a. *Often.*
   b. *Never.*
   c. *On rare occasions.*
   d. *Only when I'm drunk.*
   e. *Doesn't everybody?*

4. You find out that your fifteen-year-old daughter (sister, niece, friend) is thinking of having sex for the first time. You:

   a. *Panic.*
   b. *Ground her/tell on her.*
   c. *Sit her down for a heart-to-heart to make sure she's really ready and knows how to have safer sex.*
   d. *Sit her down for a stern lecture.*
   e. *All of the above.*

5. You're leaving a party, club, or event late at night. The friends that you came with have all left. Your car is parked several long, dark blocks away. You:

   a. *Just calmly walk to your car, taking the most lighted path available.*

b. Walk to your car as fast as you can, with your keys fanned out between your fingers and your heart pounding.

c. Ask that guy at the party who might have been flirting with you to walk you to your car.

d. Call a cab to take you to your car.

e. You would never let yourself get into that situation in the first place.

6. Women who dress and act like sluts:

a. Worry me. Don't they know the kind of attention they'll attract?

b. Make me angry. They give women a bad name and teach men they can disrespect us. They deserve whatever they get.

c. Are no better or worse than anyone else. It's not my place to judge.

d. Are powerful feminist role models. Rejecting shame about our sexuality is an act of resistance.

e. Are some of my best friends.

7. When it comes to your own sex life, you:

a. Don't have one.

b. Get exactly what you want and are totally satisfied.

c. Wish you could change a few things, but you haven't found a way to talk with your partner(s) about what you need.

d. Wish you could change a few things, but when you try to talk with your partner(s) about it, they don't respond the way you want.

e. You're not really happy with it, but you don't know what you want or how to change it.

8. Men have a harder time controlling themselves sexually and therefore can't be held to the same standards as women.

   a. *That's just biologically true.*
   b. *I'm really not sure about this one.*
   c. *That's a load of crap.*
   d. *That's true in our culture, because of the different ways we raise boys and girls.*
   e. *There may be some biological truth to that, but we're not animals—men should be expected to overcome their biological urges and control themselves.*

9. Sexual acts you do (or want to do) make you feel ashamed or bad about yourself.

   a. *All the time.*
   b. *Only one or two of them, but definitely.*
   c. *A little, maybe.*
   d. *Never.*
   e. *Almost never, but every once in a while it sneaks up on me.*

10. Your friends and family share your values about sex and sexuality.

   a. *Yes.*
   b. *My friends do, but my family really doesn't get it.*
   c. *I have no idea. I don't talk about sex with my friends or family, and they don't talk about it with me.*
   d. *Uh, no. They think I'm a total slut/prude/freak/weirdo/ etc.*
   e. *Not yet, but I'm working on them.*

Score Yourself

We're going to score this quiz a little differently than you may be used to. Instead of assigning a value to each answer, use the following as a guideline:

- If you wished any of your answers could be different than they are, this book is for you.

- If you exaggerated any of your answers in order to seem more sexually liberated/empowered/accomplished than you are, or for any other reason, this book is for you.

- If fear (possibly very valid fear) influenced any of your answers, this book is for you.

- If any of your answers reflected embarrassment or shame about sexual expression, this book is for you.

- Let's be honest. If you've read this far? This book is very likely for you.

DON'T SKIP THIS INTRODUCTION!

I remember the first time I heard the question. A reporter for a college magazine was interviewing me about *Yes Means Yes: Visions of Female Sexual Power and a World Without Rape,* the anthology I edited with Jessica Valenti. It was a long, interesting conversation about how our theories of violence prevention and sexual empowerment could be applied in real-world ways, and I was having a great time. And then she asked what now seems like the most basic question of all: Given all the conflicting messages young women get about their sexuality from all sides—media, church, family, friends, and more—how do we figure out what we want to say "yes" to in the first place?

As I struggled to form a helpful response, I thought: *Of course!* It's not like I was born with some superhuman ability to shut out a lifetime of the noise that's been thrown at me about my sexuality. Everything I now know about my own desires and boundaries has been hard-won through trial and (sometimes very unpleasant) error. And while that learning process is far from over, I do know a lot about how to figure out what I want.

I've learned that being wanted isn't the same as wanting, and it's important not to confuse the two. I've learned that I'm going to make mistakes—that just because something winds up feeling bad doesn't mean it was wrong for me to try it, as long as I tried it out of my own curiosity and not because of pressure, threats, or coercion. I've learned that direct communication is almost always the best policy, even when it feels hard or awkward, but that everyone can bring their own style to it. I've learned that there's no way to eliminate risk from my life, so the best approach is to get informed and decide which risks I'm comfortable with. I've learned that it's possible for me to violate my own boundaries, and how damaging that can be, and how to resist doing that. I've learned that love doesn't actually conquer all, even though it can be the best thing ever. I've learned that some things that are supposed to be good for me feel bad, and some things that are supposed to be bad for me feel great, and that ultimately, I get to make my own decisions about what's good and bad for me.

And that's what this book is about—equipping you to be the ultimate arbiter of what works and what doesn't work for you, sexually speaking. Because I could tell you a lot about what I really really want from my sexuality, but that's not going to tell you anything about what *you* really really want. You're the only one who can figure that out.

The good news is that you really can figure it out. You can take a long, deep look at all the voices that have shaped what you currently think about sex and figure out how to amplify the ones that work for you and turn down the ones that don't. You can learn how to evaluate risk using information and instinct and decide which risks are bogus, which risks you don't want to mess with, and which risks are real but worth taking. You can learn how to talk with partners (both present and potential) in ways that maximize pleasure and connection. You can learn how to build a sexual support group of friends who will cheer you on and check your reality when you need it, and you can learn how to deal with friends and family who may be uncomfortable with your newfound freedom. Through it all, you can reject the Terrible Trio—shame, blame, and fear—and build a sexual life that fits you so well that you find yourself humming with happiness for no apparent reason.

Sound good? It should, because it is. Sound easy? Probably not, and for good reason. The path from where you are now to where you want to end up is likely to be meandering and a little rocky. It can be uncomfortable to question things you've believed without question, and it can take time to develop faith in new ideas, even if they seem right for you. It's definitely going to require hard work, and a real commitment to yourself. But what a payoff: knowing what you really really want from sex, and knowing how to safely, sanely pursue it.

WHAT THIS BOOK WON'T DO FOR YOU

This book won't teach you how to find a boyfriend or a girl-friend. It won't offer any tips on how to make the object of your affection find you irresistible, nor will it reveal a set of rules guaranteed to get you married in under a year. Or any other amount of time.

Likewise, this book won't teach you how to "hang on" to your (wo)man, how to make a marriage last, how to keep the spark alive, or how to recapture the magic you once had.

Further, even though this is a book about sex, it won't teach you any new techniques. None. You won't learn five things guaranteed to turn a guy on, or seven sex moves guaranteed to blow her mind.

It's not that I don't know any of these things. I know a few moves that I could share, and I've learned a lot about rela-tionships and attraction over the years. But let's be honest: There's no lack of sources trying to tell you these things. If there really were definitive answers to these questions, everyone who wanted to would have a happy, hot relationship by now.

Reality is messier than that. What may attract one person can turn off another. Likewise, the sexual technique that made your ex's toes curl may make a new lover just giggle. It's a waste of time to try to learn rules that will apply to everyone. Plus, it gives your power away. Putting all of your energy into figuring out how to please or manipulate a partner makes their pleasure, their needs, and their responses more important than yours. And they're not. They're just not.

That's why this book focuses on the one sexual relationship you're going to have for your whole life: the one you have with yourself. Because once you develop a healthy, happy, reality-based relationship with your own sexuality, you'll have everything you need to figure out the rest. That doesn't mean you'll be instantly irresistible to everyone you'd ever want to attract. It may even narrow down your pool of datable prospects, not because you'll be less appealing overall (quite the opposite!), but because you'll be less appealing to people who are bad for you and you'll be less interested in them as well.

What it will do is make you more confident in your intuition about people, more appealing to people who want you exactly as you are, and more likely to have satisfying, soul- and body-fulfilling experiences with the people you do decide to be sexual with.

HOW TO USE THIS BOOK

This book isn't meant to just be read. That would put me, as the writer, in charge of telling you how to feel about your sexuality. Instead, you're in charge. Every chapter includes exercises designed to help you get to the heart of what matters most to you when it comes to sex. The exercises aren't just optional suggestions—think of each one as a rung on a ladder, or a stepping-stone on a pathway to what you really really want. They're the key to answering the questions you have about sex and unlocking a better, more authentic relationship with your own sexuality.

Each chapter is designed to be completed within a week or two, but do it at whatever pace makes the most sense for you. Don't rush—you'll get there eventually, and you'll get a lot farther if you take your time and really give the ideas and exercises the attention they require.

You may find, as you work your way through the book, that strong or surprising feelings come up for you. That's really understandable. This isn't a book about golf—it's a book about sex, one of the most powerful and elemental human experiences there is, and a subject about which many of us have painful or complex associations. There's no wrong way to feel as you do this work. We'll talk a lot more about feelings as the book goes on, but in general, please be as gentle and nonjudgmental as you can with your feelings, and ask for support from your friends, family, and/or a professional counselor as you need it.

If you're at all inclined to complete this book with a group, go for it. Gather a group of girlfriends or coworkers or cousins or whatever gang you can put together, and get together at the end of each chapter to discuss what you learned about yourself and what feelings came up for you. Not only will you learn more about each other, possibly becoming closer as a result, but you'll also feel less alone and more confident that you have compatriots who understand and support the changes you may be going through. Plus, doing the book with friends goes a long way toward keeping you on track—if you have a busy week and feel tempted to just put the book down and leave it for some other time, your group can be a great motive to keep going.

In fact, this book was developed with the help of a phenomenal crew of eleven volunteers, who experimented with each chapter in its first draft and met with me every week to talk about their experiences with sex and with the exercises. Their generous time, insight, and vulnerable honesty shaped this book in more ways than I can name, and you'll hear their voices throughout each chapter, alongside the voices of numerous other women who volunteered to share intimate details of their lives with you in order to make it possible for you to build a better, stronger sexual relationship with yourself.

That about covers everything you need to know before diving in! Are you ready to figure out what you really really want? If so, turn the page.

CHAPTER 1

YOU CAN'T GET WHAT YOU WANT TILL YOU KNOW WHAT YOU WANT

B Y THE TIME ANY OF US IS OLD ENOUGH TO THINK ABOUT sex and sexuality, we've been bombarded with so many years of confusing experiences and messages from our families, friends, culture, and media that it seems impossible to even remember that there was a time when we just knew what we wanted to do with our bodies.

Most of us can probably remember an experience when we, as kids, did something that made our bodies happy—like climbing a tree, or dressing in your mom's best silk dress because it felt good against your skin—but then learned that doing these things made other people unhappy. Or maybe you were told that doing some things that made your body happy would get you in trouble, or put you in danger—like scrambling onto the counter to reach the package of cookies your father hid on the top shelf, and then eating all of them. Maybe you learned that doing things with your body that you'd rather not do, like having to kiss your gross uncle goodbye, would make other people really happy—people you cared about, people whom you wanted to please. Or that *not* doing those things would make those people not like you anymore. This happens all the time in childhood. You're told to put your clothes back on. Go to bed when adults say so, no matter if you want to run around and play. Wear a dress, even if you want to wear pants. Don't climb that tree, you'll hurt yourself.

But instinctively knowing what feels good and what doesn't—and being able to tell other people about it—is exactly what we need to do to feel safe in our bodies and to enjoy our sexuality. So how on earth do we get there from here?

Well, I'll tell you. We can't. You read that right. The truth is, it doesn't just *feel* impossible to entirely shed the influence of the people and cultures that raised us. It *is* impossible. Even if you do everything exactly the opposite of how you were raised, you're still acting the way you are in response to those influences. None of us can ever entirely unlearn the lessons we learned growing up.

What we can do is understand those lessons. We can take a long, hard look at what messages we've absorbed about our bodies, our safety, and our sexuality; where those messages came from; and what we think about them. And, just like boosting the bass and reducing the treble on a stereo, we can decide which messages we want to amplify in our lives, and which we want to minimize. The specific balance that works for you is nobody else's business—it's the process of finding that balance that matters.

Knowing what you want from sexuality is part of knowing what you want from life. Your personal desires flow from just one emotional spigot. If you're cut off from your sexual desires, you're likely to find it much harder to know what you want in other areas of your life, whether we're talking about academics, career pursuits, or friendships.

Tuning in to what you really really want can be incredibly freeing. Not only does knowing what you want from sex significantly increase the likelihood that you'll actually get it, it's also like a love letter to yourself. Taking the time to get in touch with your own desires sends a strong message to yourself: You matter. Your opinions, instincts, beliefs, and feelings are important. You are the foremost expert about your own life and body. Paying attention to your own desires and limits teaches you to trust yourself, to be strong on your own behalf. It's a practice that can inspire you to go after what you want in all areas of your life.

In other words? Knowing what you really really want can be a heck of a lot of fun.

CLEARING A PATH

Knowing what you want and what you don't and how to act on that sounds great, doesn't it? I'll be honest—it absolutely can be. But, regardless of where you're starting from, examining your relationship with your own sexuality can be quite the journey. So, just as you would for any important trip, you've got to prepare.

Let's start with a checklist of things to do as you begin working with this book. Some of them are quick and easy, and some of them are things you'll need to keep doing the whole time you're on this journey (and may choose to keep doing even longer than that). It might be tempting to skip some, either because they seem pointless or because they seem too hard. But take it from me: The ones you want to skip are the most important ones for you to do.

Write Every Day

Starting today, and at least until you finish this book, find ten uninterrupted minutes to write every day. Doesn't matter if you like to write. Doesn't matter what you write. Doesn't matter what time of day you write. Doesn't matter if you write with pen and paper, use a keyboard, or use voice recognition software. All that matters is that you find someplace—a closet, if necessary!—where no one will disturb you for ten minutes, and that you keep writing the whole time. Write gibberish. Write, "I hate this stupid writing." Write things you've always wanted to say, or things you don't even believe. Burn or delete your writing right after you finish it if you want. Just write. And when I say "write," I don't mean "stare at the page for ten minutes and then write three sentences and call it a day." I mean write for the whole ten minutes. Your pen, your fingers on the keyboard, or your lips should not stop moving for the entire ten minutes.

But there's one stipulation! If you write a blog, or poetry, or fiction, or journalism, or anything else that is written with the expectation that someone else will read it, that doesn't count. Your ten-minute writing exercise must be independent of this.

What's with all the writing? It's simple: The process of finding your own answers to the questions this book will raise is probably going to stir up powerful feelings and thoughts for you. Imagine those feelings and thoughts are like steam, and daily writing is your release valve. It's a private place where you can say or think anything without any ramifications. Even if you're not writing about your feelings directly, it means that every day, you're taking time to listen to yourself and hear your own thoughts.

I like to do this kind of writing freehand, with a pen and paper: The physical act makes it feel immediate, and differentiates it from all the other writing that requires a keyboard. But if you prefer to use a computer, go right ahead. In fact, there are a few programs that can help you keep the words flowing. I recommend Write or Die, which forces you to keep putting words on the page for the entire ten minutes or risk virtual punishment. If you prefer a gentler approach, try Ommwriter, which helps you create a tranquil digital environment.

Not convinced? Trust me. Just do it anyway.

Note: We won't be revisiting your daily writing, but you will be doing writing exercises throughout this workbook, and you will occasionally need to refer back to the writing you do for specific exercises, so I recommend that you keep one notebook or computer folder with all your writing in it. For simplicity's sake, I'm going to tell you to "get out your notebook" by way of saying you should get in front of whatever writing system you like best.

Love Your Body

Starting now and at least until you're finished with this book, spend thirty minutes a week doing something that makes your body feel good. It doesn't have to be sexual, though it can be. However, it *must* be something you don't feel confused about. If it makes you feel good but ashamed, good but afraid, "good but . . . " anything, do something else. Maybe you'll take a bath. Maybe you'll dance or exercise. Maybe you'll slowly and deliberately eat a delicious meal. Maybe you'll get a massage. Maybe you'll masturbate. It can be a different thing each week, but it's best if it doesn't involve another person. You want to stay focused on the good feelings you're giving yourself, and not get distracted by whatever's going on with someone else. Whatever you choose to do, be sure it: (a) puts the focus on your body, and (b) makes you feel nothing but good.

Finding something to do with your body that feels good may be harder than it sounds (or maybe it doesn't sound that easy to you to begin with). As we grow up, most girls and women find it hard to avoid internalizing messages about whether or not we deserve pleasure, especially pleasure in our bodies. It's okay if this is hard—you're not alone. But you still need to do it. Start small.

> ≈≈ **Dive In:** Get out your notebook, and write down ten things that you could do to make your body feel good. Do you like the feeling of stretching? Putting moisturizer on your skin? Taking a walk? Write them down. Don't worry if you can't think of how to make a particular

activity last thirty minutes—you don't have to do the whole time all at once. Maybe instead you can spend five minutes every day luxuriously grooming your hair. You can also combine activities to make thirty minutes. The important thing is just to do it.

To get you started, here are some activities other women have tried:

- touching things that have nice textures
- playing with a pet
- walking barefoot
- painting your nails
- dancing around naked
- taking a walk in nature
- oiling your scalp
- eating something delicious
- getting extra sleep

There are a lot of good reasons to spend time giving your body pleasure on a regular basis, but there are even better reasons to make sure you do it while you're working on this book. For one, figuring out what makes you feel good is a big part of figuring out what you really really want! If you practice figuring that out in small ways every week, by the time we get to later chapters where we cover messy questions about sexual interactions with partners, you'll already have more of the skills and self-knowledge you'll need to figure out what's best for you.

It's also super likely that you've absorbed some less-than-helpful ideas about experiencing physical pleasure, and those ideas will probably get stirred up as you work your way through the book. That's natural, and this practice of loving your body can help make sure it's temporary. Practicing giving yourself pleasure will help neutralize those ideas, and maybe even replace them with some positive ideas of your own.

But the best reason of all? Because it will feel good. You never need a fancy reason to feel good.

DISCOVER WHERE YOU'RE STARTING FROM

Ready for another quiz? I thought so. This one's designed to help you get a handle on where you're at on the journey to knowing and getting what you really really want. Like the first one, we're not going to score it. Instead, you'll take it again when you're done with this book, to help you see the ways in which you've developed.

So get out a pen, and get answering: There's no way to do it wrong.

1. I know how to stay safe while expressing my sexuality.

   Strongly Disagree   ① ② ③ ④ ⑤ ⑥ ⑦ ⑧ ⑨ ⑩   *Strongly Agree*

2. I'm afraid of what others would think/say/do if they knew how I felt about sex.

   Strongly Disagree   ① ② ③ ④ ⑤ ⑥ ⑦ ⑧ ⑨ ⑩   *Strongly Agree*

3. I can tell when sexual activity is making me uncomfortable.

   Strongly Disagree   ① ② ③ ④ ⑤ ⑥ ⑦ ⑧ ⑨ ⑩   *Strongly Agree*

4. I can tell when sexual activity is giving me pleasure.

Strongly Disagree ① ② ③ ④ ⑤ ⑥ ⑦ ⑧ ⑨ ⑩ *Strongly Agree*

5. I feel comfortable telling a potential sexual partner that something they're doing is making me uncomfortable.

Strongly Disagree ① ② ③ ④ ⑤ ⑥ ⑦ ⑧ ⑨ ⑩ *Strongly Agree*

6. I feel comfortable telling a potential sexual partner what to do in order to give me pleasure.

Strongly Disagree ① ② ③ ④ ⑤ ⑥ ⑦ ⑧ ⑨ ⑩ *Strongly Agree*

7. My beliefs and attitudes about sex make sense to me.

Strongly Disagree ① ② ③ ④ ⑤ ⑥ ⑦ ⑧ ⑨ ⑩ *Strongly Agree*

8. I often do sexual things or have sexual feelings that make me feel confused or bad.

Strongly Disagree ① ② ③ ④ ⑤ ⑥ ⑦ ⑧ ⑨ ⑩ *Strongly Agree*

9. My sexual partner(s), if I have them, share my beliefs and attitudes about sex.

Strongly Disagree ① ② ③ ④ ⑤ ⑥ ⑦ ⑧ ⑨ ⑩ *Strongly Agree*

10. My friends share my beliefs and attitudes about sex.

Strongly Disagree ① ② ③ ④ ⑤ ⑥ ⑦ ⑧ ⑨ ⑩ *Strongly Agree*

11. My family shares my beliefs and attitudes about sex.

Strongly ① ② ③ ④ ⑤ ⑥ ⑦ ⑧ ⑨ ⑩ *Strongly*
Disagree   *Agree*

12. I have people in my life I feel comfortable talking to about sex.

Strongly ① ② ③ ④ ⑤ ⑥ ⑦ ⑧ ⑨ ⑩ *Strongly*
Disagree   *Agree*

Make a Commitment

The last and possibly most important thing on your checklist has to do with getting clear about why you're engaging with this book at all. That may seem like a big "duh" to you. You may have picked up this book for a very explicit reason, like: "I want to be able to talk to my partner about how to make sex better for me." Or it may seem like a tall order. Maybe you're still not sure why you're doing this at all. Maybe it's just a gut feeling you're following. Maybe you've picked up this book because a friend wants you to work on it with her.

The thing is, some of what we're going to cover in this book is going to feel difficult. I can't tell you which parts of the book you'll have reactions to—it's going to be different for everyone. But odds are, at least one or two sections are going to be hard enough that you feel like giving up. You may think, *This is hard and stupid and pointless. Why am I even bothering?*

That's why it's so important to take some time right now, before you begin, to think about what you want to get out of this book. Perhaps the "Discover Where You're Starting From" quiz can guide you—wish any of your responses could change?

There's no right answer to the question of what you want from this process—only *your* answer (or answers!). The crucial thing is to get as clear as you can about it now and then write it down, so that when you get lost or confused or frustrated or pissed off or whatever, you can go back and read what you wrote now and help yourself stay on track to getting what you need.

> **Dive In:** Send yourself a message. Using your notebook or recording to audio or video, send your future self a message about why you're committing to this process, what you want to get out of it, and what you want your future self to remember when things start to feel hard. Say whatever you want, but also be sure to include the following sentences: "I, [your name], am making a promise to myself: I won't quit this process. I'm starting it for a reason, and I'll see it through to the end. Because I matter to myself. My desires matter, my pleasure matters, and my safety matters. What I really really want matters. This process is a gift to myself, and I promise to accept it."
>
> Feel silly writing or saying some of these things? Not sure if you mean them? That's okay. Do it anyway.

INFLUENCES

All right. Now that you've committed yourself to discovering what you really really want, it's time to start the process of figuring out just that. But before we start finding a good path forward for you, we have to spend some time figuring out where you've come from and where you are now. Let's start by taking a look at the forces that have influenced your beliefs about sex

so far. As we do this, remember the stereo equalizer: The goal
here isn't to remove these influences—that wouldn't be possible
even if you wanted to. The goal is to figure out which of these
influences you want to turn up the volume on, and which ones
you want to minimize.

*(A note on influences: Not all of us have been strongly influ-
enced by all of the following common influences. Some of us
weren't raised with a religion; others of us were homeschooled.
If you feel a particular influence hasn't applied to you at all, feel
free to skip it.)*

Family

It's hard to talk about families in a general way, because every
family is different. That's not just some *Sesame Street* lesson—it's
hard to think of another social structure that's so important and
yet so hard to define. "Families" are made up of a wide variety of
different kinds and combinations of people. Different "families"
have vastly different values from each other, and very different
ideas about what a "family" is, and what it's for. Some people's
families are incredibly loving, open, supportive, creative communities. Some people's families are abusive, poisonous nightmares.
Some people don't grow up with a family at all. Most of us have
flawed but well-meaning families—there may be some messed-
up dynamics present, but everybody's doing their best with what
they've got, and hopefully the good stuff outweighs the bad.

One of the few things most families have in common is
that the people in your family are the first folks to teach you
what you should and shouldn't do with your body. It starts the

moment you're born, and for most families doesn't stop, well, ever. Maybe they tell you to eat your broccoli because it will give you energy. Maybe they stop you from putting your finger in an electrical outlet, because they know that, sometimes, keeping you safe is more important than indulging your curiosity. Families are almost always where you find the primary adults who shape your life as you grow up and try to figure out the world. They've had bodies a lot longer than you have, and they have a lot of ideas about what to do with them. In short: They think they know better than you. And a lot of times, like when it comes to broccoli and electrical sockets, they're right.

But when it comes to what you should do with your body sexually, families can get *complicated*. Your family may have very strong beliefs about sex—beliefs that they may expect you to abide by, whether or not you really agree with them. Heck, they may not even agree with each other, or with their own relatives, about what's right and wrong when it comes to sex. Even more likely, your family may say little or nothing to you directly about sexuality, but instead convey their beliefs through the way they treat you and your body: stuff like offhand comments about your clothes, rules about what parts of your body are okay for you or other people to touch, assumptions about who you might be attracted to, or how you might behave around people you're attracted to—you get the idea.

Take twenty-four-year-old Gray, for example, who says she grew up in a very religious family: "I was taught that my body was something to hide from men—including male members of my family. And I was always so confused about why I couldn't sleep in the basement with my cousin when we were twelve, and why I had to be hyperconscious of it when I was walking around the house."

Jill, twenty-seven, had a much different experience.

My parents raised me to feel full ownership over my body, including my sexuality, by encouraging me to use my body in productive, pleasure-centered ways that weren't necessarily sexual. I grew up playing sports, sharing healthy and delicious family meals, being sent to arts camp, and going biking and camping and skiing with my family on the weekends and for vacations. My parents also talked to me about the birds and the bees and left a copy of Our Bodies, Ourselves around, and my mom was clear that if I ever needed birth control I could ask the doctor and it would be totally confidential—and all of those things were great—but the best thing my parents did to help me develop a healthy view of sex was to encourage me to own my body and to use it in ways that felt good.

And what your family teaches you directly is only part of the equation. We learn so much from watching how the people around us behave, and our families are often the people around us the most as we're growing up. If you watch members of your family be abusive or shaming or hurtful to each other, you're going to absorb different lessons than if you watch your family be loving and supportive and respectful about sexuality.

The thing is, whatever your family's attitudes about sexuality, they didn't get those values from nowhere. They've been influenced by the same forces that influence all of us: the media, their own family and friends, their religious beliefs, what they were taught in school, etc. And they may never have examined their beliefs about sex as thoroughly as someone like you, who's picked up this here fine book.

All of which is to say: Just because your family believes certain things about sex or acts certain ways—even if they seem really sure about what they believe or how they act—doesn't mean those beliefs are right for you. In order to figure out what you really really want, you've got to think about the lessons you've learned from your family and decide what you value and what you might want to let go of in order to move forward with what you want.

Dive In: Write a short paragraph beginning with each of the following phrases:

- When it comes to sex and sexuality, my family _____

- My family's attitudes about sexuality have been influenced by _____

- Something my family taught me about sexuality that I agree with is _____

- Something my family taught me about sexuality that I disagree with is _____

- Something my family taught me about sexuality that I'm confused or unsure about is _____

- When I disagree with my family about sexuality, they _____

Media

Is there any more confusing source of information about sexuality than the media? Whether it's the movies or TV, video games or the nightly news, music or gossip websites—to say nothing of porn—sexual images of women are everywhere in our mass media. But what do they tell us?

On the one hand, if you went by the mass media, you'd think that it was a legal requirement that all girls and women look sexy at all times, and a very particular kind of sexy at that: perfect hair, polished nails, shaved legs, trendy clothes, etc. Not to mention white, thin, able-bodied, young, and conventionally pretty. In medialand, if you fail to do and be all of these things, you're either evil or pathetic or both. But look *too* sexy—wear too much makeup, clothes too short or too tight, etc.—or act like you actually want sex too much, and you're a "slut," which also makes you evil or pathetic or both.

That teeny window of "correct" female sexuality in the media is a big tip-off that something's wrong. There are so many different kinds of women, and we experience our sexualities a million different ways—sometimes all on the same day. So if the media are showing only one (or even two or three!) of those ways, they're clearly not trying to represent the experiences of real women. But what *are* they trying to do?

Mostly, they're trying to sell stuff. TV shows want you to buy whatever their advertisers are selling, so the companies will keep advertising and the show can stay on the air. Movies are trying to sell tickets and DVDs. Video games are selling not just the game itself, but the next version of the game (which is always coming out soon!), the merch associated with it, etc.

You get the picture. Whatever the medium, one of the most popular ways of trying to sell us stuff is by presenting impossibly narrow and idealized representations of women.

What's that do? Well, it tells women that they can be happy, but only if they buy the infinite things required to make them look and act like the media's Ideal Woman. And it tells (straight) men that they can be happy, but only if they buy the infinite things required to attract the media's Ideal Woman.

To make matters worse, our mass media often treats violence against women casually (think *Grand Theft Auto*) or like a joke (as in the movie *Observe and Report*), and passive, normative women's sexuality (think the Victoria's Secret fashion show) like wholesome entertainment, while treating complex and authentic portrayals of sex as beyond the pale and dangerous to minors. Is it any wonder we live in such a violent and sexually repressed culture, or that we're deeply and often permanently confused about the many ways we deviate from those artificial ideals?

Dive In: Think back to some adolescent media crushes—that song or album you listened to over and over, the magazine subscription you thought would change your life, the book you picked up again and again, the movie you imagined yourself starring in, the video game you played and played and played, the TV show you just couldn't miss. What drew you to these particular experiences? What, if anything, did they say to you about sexuality? What lessons did you learn from them that you've since rejected, and what did you learn that you still adhere to today? If you could go back and tell your adolescent self something about your media choices, what would it be? Get out your journal, and write about it for five minutes.

Peers

Let's face it: As much as we like to see ourselves as independent thinkers, it can matter a lot what people think of us. So your peers' attitudes toward sex and sexuality are probably going to have a big impact on you, for better or for worse.

This influence can work a lot of different ways. Some of them have to do with comparing your sexual behavior to other people's: Maybe everyone you know is having sex or doing some particular sex act and thinks you're weird because you don't want to, or aren't ready, or haven't found the right circumstances for you. Maybe the opposite is true—you're sexually active in a way that no one around you seems to be, and you feel like you can't say anything about it, or they'll think you're bad, amoral, or "easy."

Twenty-four-year-old Zeinab shares how she struggled with this: "A few of my friends are very conservative, and when I started exploring more of my sexuality and sharing that with them, a lot of times I felt like I was getting veiled hostility, and I felt like I was getting shamed by them as well, because they weren't doing what I was doing, and so it almost felt like they were acting superior to me."

Sometimes peer attitudes about sexuality come out in ways that have nothing to do with what sexual activities you are or aren't participating in. If you've been teased for being "slutty" or "trampy" or a "ho," it's probably not because the people doing the teasing (who, let's face it, are just as likely to be other girls as they are to be boys) have information about what you're doing sexually. More likely, it's because you dress differently, or exhibit a kind of confidence in your body other girls don't, or even simply because you're unafraid to express your opinion about things that have nothing to do with sex. The exact same things can be said for girls who are accused of being "dykes" or "lesbians"—those "accusations" rarely have anything to do with actual sexual orientation, and everything to do with the insecurities and immaturities of the people using those words.

Sexuality-related judgments are used all the time to police not-very-sexual behaviors, because they work. For most of us, those kinds of pronouncements cut close to the bone, because there can be very real consequences to being seen as a "slut" or a "dyke." There's not anything actually wrong with being a woman who has a lot of sex or a woman who is sexually attracted to other women, but those kinds of labels can be used to excuse taunting, shaming, social excommunication, and even violence.

Fortunately, peers can also be an enormous support when it comes to navigating your sexuality. Good friends—ones who support your happiness and health, whatever form it takes—can be great sounding boards when you're experimenting with new ideas or experiences. They can be your lead cheerleaders when you're setting difficult boundaries with yourself or other people.

They can laugh with you (not at you!) about how ridiculous all this sex stuff is sometimes. They can comfort you if you're grappling with trauma or heartbreak. They can be incredible resources when you're looking for ideas, information, advice, or reality checks. And they can defend you and reassure you when it seems like other people are judging you for your sexual choices.

Shira, age nineteen, learned this the best way. "While so many of my friends were telling me to read *Cosmo* articles as preparation for my first time having sex," she remembers, "one friend talked to me instead about masturbation, finding my clitoris, and instructing my partner. She taught me to be my own first partner. For her, I am so grateful."

That's why it's important to be choosy about your friends.

Dive In: Actually, this is more of a "don't do this." As you embark on this journey, be cautious about who you discuss it with. Even good friends of yours may be challenged by hearing about the questions you're now asking yourself and the things you're learning. This can happen even with friends who truly have your best interest at heart, because hearing about the issues you're grappling with might remind them of how uncomfortable they themselves feel with their own sexuality, and how little they know what they really really want. It's natural to want to talk about this process and the strong feelings it's probably going to bring up, but the best thing to do is to share those feelings with a friend who's taking the journey with you. If you don't have a partner in this process,

see if you can find someone to confide in whose relationship with her sexuality you admire. Above all, remember:
If people are making you feel bad about engaging in this
process, that's telling you something about them, not anything about you. Don't go back to those people for support on these issues.

School

What did you learn about sexuality in school? If you're like
most students in the United States, you probably learned that
sex is both emotionally and physically dangerous if you have
it before you're married. If you're "lucky," you then learned
how to prevent some of the greatest risks of sex, just in case
you were going to insist on doing it anyhow. If you weren't as
lucky (if you were the beneficiary, for example, of U.S. federal
initiatives in the last decade that poured more than a billion dollars into sex education programs that taught abstinence as the
only choice), you likely learned that girls who have sex before
marriage are like presucked candy, have given away the most
precious thing they have to someone who doesn't deserve it, or
are just plain doomed to hell.

There's a reason, of course, that schools teach this way—
they're made up of people who've grown up in our messed-up sexual culture, and they're trying teach what they can while offending
the fewest people possible. But the problem with both of these
approaches is that they treat sex like a yes-or-no question—and
one with only one correct answer at that. The reality is much
more complicated. (You probably already know that on some

level, or you wouldn't be reading this book.) Sexuality encompasses a vast spectrum of feelings, thoughts, and desires, none of which are "wrong" or "right" so much as they just *are*. It's what you do with them that matters. As long as what you do with your sexuality (a) doesn't hurt anyone else and (b) doesn't hurt you or expose you to unnecessary risk (we'll be talking lots more about how to decide what risks are unnecessary in chapter 4), then there is literally nothing you can do that's actually "wrong."

I'll say that again because it bears repeating: As long as you're not hurting anyone (including yourself), then there is *no wrong way* to express or experience your sexuality.

The problem is, that's a complex statement. What does it mean to hurt someone else, or yourself, with your sexuality? How can you tell if you're hurting someone or yourself? And if there's no wrong way, that leaves open a dizzying variety of options that can feel overwhelming and hard to navigate. Helping you sort it all out is one of the main purposes of this book. But this book might not even be necessary if, instead of spending all that time telling you that "giving it away" too soon was the worst decision you could make with your life, schools spent time actually helping you figure out what kinds of sexual expression and experience were right for you. What if they'd taught you how to make your own informed, healthy decisions about sex? And what if you could assume that nearly everyone else you might want to interact with sexually had had the same lessons?

School is also a place where many of us experience physical violations in "small" ways—think bra snapping, butt grabbing, and the like—and school is far too often a place where we learn that, even if we complain, boys are given blanket permission to violate our boundaries in these ways. This "boys will be boys" mentality leads to what I call the "boiling frog" problem of women's sexual boundaries. I call it that because of the legend that if you put a frog into a pot of boiling water, it will jump right out, but if you put a frog into a pot of room-temperature water and slowly heat it to a boil, the frog will acclimate as the water heats up and never jump out, eventually boiling to death. Similarly, when we learn as young girls to tolerate "low-level" boundary violations like the ones we often are forced to suffer in silence at school, it makes it harder for us to notice when even greater boundaries are being violated, eventually leading to the reality that many women who are pressured into having sex against their will don't even recognize it as a form of violence (though that lack of naming hardly spares them the trauma of the experience). On the other hand, schools that teach, through actions as well as policy, that everyone has a right to their own boundaries and no one has the right to touch you in ways that you don't like are teaching girls to recognize and name it if they ever find themselves in really hot water.

Dive In: Make a list of everything your schools have taught you about sexuality. Now make another list, of at least five things you wish they had taught you but didn't. Now pick one thing on that second list you still wish you knew more about, and go to Scarleteen.com—a fantastic site about sexuality—and read up on it.

RELIGIOUS INSTITUTIONS

If you were raised in any kind of religious tradition, odds are, you were taught some very particular sexual values (that is, a set of beliefs about what's right and wrong when it comes to sex) in conjunction with that faith. And depending on how you feel about the rest of your religion, you may put more or less stock in those dictates about sexuality.

I'm not going to waste your time summarizing the way different religions think about sex—it would be almost as foolish as trying to list all the different ways families think about sex. Even within any given religion, there are subgroups that vary widely on their approach to the matter. Besides, all that really counts is what your religion has taught you. And you know that better than I do.

Honestly, the religion-family analogy is pretty strong when it comes to sex, the main difference being what's at stake. If you go against your family's values when it comes to sex, you might be grounded or otherwise punished by your family. In extreme cases, your family may be violent to you, or kick you out of the house, or disown you. That's all pretty awful. But religion has bigger weapons still, depending on what faith you belong to. Your religion may tell you that if you stray from its sexual principles, you'll suffer for all eternity. Some fundamentalist religions believe that women who violate their sexual norms should be publicly shamed, or even killed. The fear these threats instill can make it difficult to even question what your religion has taught you about women and sex. But you're not alone, and you're obviously up to the challenge, or you wouldn't be reading this paragraph.

The other things to think about when it comes to sex and your religion are these questions: Why does my religion teach me these things about sex? What is my religion's attitude toward women's equality in general? Some—though certainly not all— religions believe that men should be dominant over women, and they use their sexual teachings to keep women afraid and compliant with a system that doesn't have their best interests at heart. If you can think about your religion's sexual teachings as part of its values about women in general, it may help you see what drives those teachings, and whether or not you want to learn from them.

Dive In: Complete the following sentences. If you've received conflicting religious messages about sex, feel free to choose the ones that seem loudest or strongest to you:

- When it comes to sex, my religion tells me

  _____

- One thing my religion says about sex that I agree with is _____

- One thing my religion says about sex that I disagree with is _____

- One thing my religion says about sex that I have questions about is _____

- If I don't act the way my religion says I should sexually, I've been taught that _____

Medical Professionals

Because doctors, nurses, and therapists are the people we turn to when we need expert advice about our bodies and minds, they can have an incredible influence on how we understand our sexuality. But for better and for worse, our medical professionals are also influenced by all of the factors we've been discussing in this chapter, so they can promote harmful stereotypes just as easily as they can provide helpful information.

Prerna, twenty-three, shares her experience with this. "As a sex-positive teen, I went to my first gynecologist appointment with lots of questions about safety and health. But I never asked any of them, because one of the first things the doctor asked me was if I was having intercourse, and when I told her I wasn't, she looked at me like I was lying and asked me again. It went well beyond 'you can trust me and should be honest' and was definitely more of 'we all know you're a slut, so just admit it.' It freaked me out because I really wasn't expecting virgin shame from my doctor, of all people."

Shana, twenty-eight, had a similar experience. "I stopped anwering their questions truthfully when at a more recent visit they asked me how many sex partners I had in the last year, and when I answered honestly, they gave me a twenty-minute safe-sex talk. They never even asked me if I was having safe sex, or if I knew how to. I'm known amongst my friends for always, always having condoms with me and handing them out to unprepared friends."

And it's not just in terms of the virgin/slut dichotomy that medical professionals can fail. Some therapists have been known to blame victims for their sexual assault, and doctors may make false and silencing assumptions about the gender of your sexual partners. Pharmacists have denied birth control[1] (and even, in a 2011 case, lifesaving antibleeding medication[2]) to women because they disapproved of those women's sexual choices, and doctors all over regularly deny women the information they need to get an abortion, which is a safe and legal procedure in the United States. The list goes on.

On the other hand, some medical professionals can be lifesavers, giving you information and access to sexual health care that your family or community may make difficult to get, and otherwise supporting your healthy pursuit of what you really really want. My current doctor, for example, supports my efforts to love and accept my body by practicing medicine from a Health at Every Size perspective. That means she may tell me I should eat healthier and exercise more because my cholesterol is too high, but she'll never tell me I need to lose weight, because she knows that the scale tells you nothing about a person's health.[3] And my therapist supports my sexual decisions as long as they seem to be coming from a healthy and centered place—even when those decisions find me having casual, safe sex with strangers.

The psychological and practical power medical professionals can have on our sexuality is profound indeed, which is why it's really important to examine what we've already learned from medical experts we've encountered—and also to find providers in the present tense whose values support our own.

This can be a challenge, depending on where you live and how much money or medical insurance you have access to. But there are resources for finding truly helpful medical care. One of them is Scarleteen's Find-a-Doc service, where you can recommend healthcare providers you've had positive experiences with, and get recommendations from others if you need to find someone better or new. Find-a-Doc covers not only doctors, but also counselors, LGBTQ centers, doulas, shelters, and other in-person sexual/reproductive health, sexuality, and/or crisis care. Share your tips or find ones from others at www.wyrrw.com/scarleteenfindadoc.

Dive In: Get out your journal, and write for five to ten minutes about an experience you've had with a medical professional that influenced your sexuality. Maybe it was a scary or negative experience, or maybe it was a positive, empowering one. What did the person do or say that made an impact? What did you learn from them? How did you respond? Do you still believe in that lesson today? Why or why not?

Partners

If you've already been sexually active with a partner, or even if you've just experienced strong desire for a particular person, you know just how much that person can influence how you feel about your sexuality.

The tricky part here is that it's hard to control who you want, and yet wanting someone sexually makes their opinion of you seem important. That can be wonderful: There are few better feelings than having your desires reciprocated. It can make you feel all kinds of good things: desired, loved, beautiful, strong. And being sexually open with someone can strengthen the bonds of intimacy in many ways, leaving us feeling safe and understood and supported.

But sexual partners can also have the opposite effect. They can leave us feeling inadequate or like freaks. They can pressure us to want things we don't want, and do things we don't want to do. Or they can make us feel bad about the desires we do have, or the sexual interactions we've already experienced. They can abuse us physically or mentally, and they can use our desire for them to control us, leaving us feeling that our very desire is dangerous to us.

Dive In: Make a list of five sexual partners you've had or wished you could have. Don't worry about how you choose them; just write down the first five that come to mind. Now, for each of them, answer the following questions: How do you feel about your sexuality when you think about them? Did/do they try to give you what you want/ed sexually? Did/do they ever make you feel bad about your sexuality? Did/do they make you feel safe, or loved or scared or abused, or all of the above?

It's beyond fine to be influenced by other people and institutions—it's unavoidable. But you have more choice than you may have known when it comes to how much and in what ways you're influenced. This chapter is a great start—but don't stop now. Adjust the balance levels over time, so that the sound you're getting gets closer and closer to the ideal soundtrack to accompany you on this journey to what you really really want.

Dive In: Make a life chart on a large piece of paper (landscape view). Draw a line across the paper horizontally. Then divide your age by five, and divide the line into five equal sections, each representing a fifth of how long you've been alive. (So, if you're twenty-five years old, divide the line into five-year segments, from birth to five years old, five to ten, etc.) For each section, write at least one key incident that happened in that period that shaped your attitudes or feelings about your sexuality—from a video to a favorite song, to something your parents told you (that either did or didn't match up with the way they behaved), to whatever you were taught in school, to actual sexual experiences you or your friends had that have made an impact. Don't worry about getting everything down right now—we'll be filling in this timeline throughout the process of this book.

Now choose one of these incidents and write about where you were (the location), who was there (the characters), and what happened (the incident). You can do this for any or all of the incidents you have listed.

Go Deeper: At the end of every chapter, you'll find a few optional exercises that you can use to go deeper into the process of this book. The best ones to choose are the ones that provoke a strong reaction when you read them—even if it's that you think you'll hate doing it.

1. Stick a photograph of yourself (one you like) in your journal. Write the woman in the photograph a love letter. List all the things she does well or that you like about her.

2. If you could take yourself on a date, where would it be? What would you do? Describe your perfect date in detail.

3. Keep a media journal. This week, pay attention to the depictions of women's sexuality you see in the media. Think about what song lyrics are saying, how billboards are pairing women and sex, what the characters in your favorite TV shows and video games act like (and what the consequences of those actions are), how the women in the books, newspapers, magazines, and websites you read are portrayed, etc. At the end of every day, write down what you remember and how those depictions made you feel. And at the end of the week, make a list of which media outlets gave you mostly positive feelings, which were mostly negative, and which were a mixed bag.

CHAPTER 2

BAD THINGS COME IN THREES: SHAME, BLAME, AND FEAR

EVERYWHERE I GO, WHENEVER I TALK ABOUT SEX AND rape and how women should have just as much right as men to pursue sexual pleasure on their own terms, I hear the same question coming from the women in the audience. It's a very sincere and urgent question, and it breaks my heart every time I hear it: *But how do I even know what I want?*

That question haunts me because in an ideal world it would never even be asked. In a better world, it wouldn't be that hard to *know* what we want, sexually or otherwise. We would be able to tell by what *felt* good. (Radical idea, huh?) Just as there are forces in the world influencing how we *perceive* our sexuality, which we explored in chapter 1, these same forces can work against us in other ways, in an effort to *control* our behavior.

Sometimes it's the media, trying to sell us something. Sometimes it's our families, friends, or partners, who want us to behave in ways that make them more happy or comfortable, even if it makes us unhappy, uncomfortable, or worse. Sometimes it's a religious or political faction that believes women should be subservient to men.

Whoever it is, whatever the motives are behind their actions, the methods they use are always the same: shame, blame, and fear. They're telling us that we should be ashamed of our sexuality or that our sexual desires and actions are to blame for outcomes that aren't actually our fault (such as sexual assault) or that if we pursue what we want sexually, we'll be in danger (of getting a disease, of violence, of never finding love, you name it), so we should be wary of expressing our sexuality, or even outright afraid of it.

When you're controlled by the Terrible Trio, as I like to call the triple threat of shame, blame, and fear, bad things happen. For one, you just feel crappy about yourself—second-guessing your decisions, worrying how people see you, feeling responsible for everything—and that crappy feeling can lead to even crappier outcomes. For example, if you feel insecure about your sexuality, you often don't want to associate with your desires. You end up checking out of your body a little, like you're watching yourself in a movie. In that checked-out state, whatever sexual encounters you engage in can feel like they "just happen" to you. You might have unprotected sex because you're too afraid to admit to yourself that you want to have sex at all to speak up about using barriers. Or, if you're "just letting" someone make out with you (because you secretly want to make out with them but you're in denial about it), you might wind up "just letting" them do sexual things with you that you really don't want as well. All of these dynamics collide to create one massive negative-feedback loop in which you feel bad about sex, which makes sex feel bad, which makes you feel even worse about it.

On the other hand, if you find ways to reject the Terrible Trio, you can create the exact opposite effect: You'll feel more connected to your sexuality, which means it will be easier for you to get your sexual needs met, which will feel great, which will make you feel even better about your sexuality.

SHAME

Odds are, at some point, someone has tried to make you feel ashamed of your sexuality. Maybe someone, a parent or a classmate, said you were dressed "slutty." Maybe you told a date you didn't want to be sexual, or even just be sexual in a particular way, and they called you "uptight" or a "prude." Or maybe the opposite happened, and you expressed your sexuality openly and with exuberance, and you were suddenly labeled "easy." It doesn't have to be about your behavior, either. You could feel shamed by something as simple as what arouses you. Take twenty-six-year-old Avory, for example. "My most sensitive spot is just under my armpit, which I find very, very embarrassing and often can't even admit, because it seems so nonstandard and armpits are 'icky.'"

Often, this shame gets lodged in our bodies. We feel ashamed of how we look, or we feel ashamed of how others see

us, or we feel ashamed of what gives us physical pleasure and
what doesn't.

The variations on the shame theme are endless. But shame
always boils down to one thing: A person or group is projecting
their moral values onto you. It doesn't even have to be directly
targeted at you. Twenty-one-year-old Mag puts it best here:

*The way my friends or people around me talk about expe-
riences they've had with people, and the way Cosmo is
constantly like, "50 ways to please your man" and, "OMG,
virgins," it makes me feel ashamed to not have had these
experiences. And it makes it even harder for me to get
out there and tell somebody, because I'm afraid that once
they know that I haven't done certain things, they're not
going to want to do that with me, because they'll think
there must be something wrong with me.*

When someone is making you feel ashamed about your
behavior, your appearance, or anything, for that matter, the
most important thing to ask yourself is: Do I agree with this
person's values?

This seems like a pretty easy thing to do, but in practice it's
actually pretty complex, especially when you're not in the habit
of asking yourself the question in the first place, and particularly when you haven't asked yourself the corollary question:
What are my personal values about sexuality?

This is a good place for me to own up to my own values
around sex, but let me be the first to say: You don't have to

agree with me! The important thing is to spend the time deciding for *yourself* what you believe.

I believe that we all have the right to experience sexual pleasure. For the vast majority of us,[1] sexuality is a central part of our humanity, a basic pleasure, like enjoying the taste of food or laughing until we cry. On a more practical level, if it makes me feel good before, during, and after; and if it involves other people and makes *them* feel good before, during, and after; *and* if everyone understands the risks involved and takes reasonable precautions to be safe, then, well, what's not to like? For example, if you and your partner both love giving and receiving oral sex, then by all means, enjoy it with abandon. It's really that simple, yet the Terrible Trio has any number of powerful ways to make you feel that it's a shameful, even disgusting, taboo.

Of course, much of this is also open to interpretation. For example, what's a "risk," and what's "reasonable"? For that matter, what's "safe"? And how do you know if your partner is feeling good? These are valid questions, but none of them have simple answers. We'll continue to address them as we make our way through this journey together.

But remember, whether you agree or disagree with my values, what matters is that you know what your *own* values are. Once you know what you believe about sexuality, you build up an immunity to shame. How? Just do your best to act according to your beliefs. (Hint: If that seems impossible, you may want to check in with yourself to make sure your values are realistic and allow for you to be a messy, complicated person. Because we're all messy and complicated at least some of the time.)

If you know what your sexual values are and adhere to them most of the time, then it's going to be a lot harder for other people to make you feel shame.

> **Dive In:** Write a sexual mission statement. This should be a paragraph expressing what you believe about sexuality. Be sure to answer the following questions: What do you have the right to, sexually? What are your responsibilities when it comes to sex? What about your partners' rights and responsibilities? What's the most important thing you seek from sexual exploration or expression? What do you never want to seek from sexuality? What does no one have the right to do when it comes to sex?
>
> Now, write a list of five times you've felt sex-related shame. Circle two of those five that felt particularly intense. Then pick one, and write out the story of what happened—what did you do or not do that triggered the shame? Did someone try to shame you for it directly, or did the shame come from the inside, from something you'd previously absorbed? Describe the shame you felt as specifically as you can. Now read back over your sexual mission statement, and apply it to this situation. Do you now, in the present tense, think you did anything wrong then?

BLAME

Oy. Blame. What hasn't been blamed on female sexuality? When women act on behalf of our own sexual desires, we get blamed for being raped, for the demise of modern masculinity, for men's cheating, for getting cervical cancer, for homophobia, for street harassment, even for earthquakes. But the truth is, there are very few ways to hurt yourself, your partner, or society through your sexuality.

Here's the complete list of things that you should worry about during sex:

- Are my partner and I both enthusiastic about what's happening, and both capable of free and enthusiastic consent? (More on enthusiastic consent in chapter 7.)

- Are we taking reasonable precautions to prevent STDs and other bodily harm?

- If, between us, we've got the physical equipment required to make a baby, are we using a reliable form of birth control, or do we both want a pregnancy?

That's it. That's the whole list. If you've got those bases covered, and you're not lying to any of your partners, and you're not an adult who's cheating or willingly committing incest, I guarantee you're not doing anything wrong.

So why are there so many bad behaviors that get blamed on women's sexuality? That's a great question, and sometimes we have to recognize when and where it's happening so we can understand that we're not at fault, and how to redirect that blame so it lands where it belongs—which is on the perpetrators of the behaviors, not on us.

Street Harassment

Say you wake up one morning feeling kinda sexy. Maybe you had a great sexual encounter the night before. Maybe your new workout routine is giving you great energy. Maybe it's spring and the warm air is making you feel tingly. So you go to your closet and put on something that suits your mood. Maybe it's a little clingy, or swingy, or the fabric feels great. Maybe it shows off your shoulders or your legs or your cleavage.

So, you're walking down the street, feeling hot, having a great day, and suddenly you hear him. From a car, perhaps, or maybe just from across the street. He's yelling gross comments at you, or making rude gestures. It could be anything from, "Nice tits, baby," with accompanying hand gestures to illustrate what he'd like to do to them, to the vile thing my friend Chloe, age twenty-three, heard when she was walking down the street one day: "Damn, baby, I wanna put you in a cage!"

If you asked this guy why he's shouting at you, he'd probably tell you that (a) he meant it as a compliment, and (b) if you didn't want the attention, you shouldn't have dressed so sexy.

"If she's a slut, you have to treat her like a slut" is what one young street harasser told reporter Joe Eaton at the *Washington City Paper* in a story on the phenomenon.[2] But street harassment isn't your fault, no matter what you wear—and it has little to do with your wardrobe.

As much as harassers want to claim their behavior is sexually motivated, the truth is, it's really about power. When I get harassed on the street, it usually has less to do with what I'm wearing and more to do with how I'm feeling. Most of the time, creeps target me when I'm feeling tired or nervous or lost or distracted, not when I'm feeling confident and strong. It's got nothing to do with what I'm wearing or how "good" I look. And I'm not alone. When Jezebel.com surveyed its readers about what they were doing when they were harassed on the street, the three most popular answers by far were: minding my own business, wearing jeans, and having no makeup on.[3]

It's important to recognize that however we feel about the harassment ourselves, it's still not our fault. Some women, like twenty-six-year-old Becca, sometimes find themselves struggling with conflicted responses: "I have, at times, felt like it was simultaneously really affirming of my femininity, and really awful from a political standpoint."

There's nothing wrong or surprising about that—of course all of us have been exposed to the myth that any male attention should be taken as a compliment, and that vulnerability is a valued feminine characteristic. None of these feelings mean you've "asked for it" or are "bringing it on yourself."

There's a growing movement of women who recognize that street harassment isn't our fault and are doing something about it. They're reporting harassers online and to the authorities, snapping pictures with their cell phones, sometimes even confronting them in the moment. What all of these women have in common is that they are placing the blame where it belongs: not on their own behaviors, but on their harassers'. For their inspiring stories, and resources that you can use in your own life, check out ihollaback.org.

Couples Harassment

If you walk down the street holding your female partner's hand, or kiss her in public, or even just look "dykey" together (or by yourself), some Neanderthals may decide to yell at you, threaten you, or hurt you. That's awful, and it's also a hate crime in

the United States and many other countries. (U.S. federal law
permits federal prosecution of anyone who "willingly injures,
intimidates or interferes with another person, or attempts to do
so, by force because of the other person's race, color, religion,
national origin, actual or perceived gender, sexual orientation,
gender identity, or disability.")[4] But one thing it isn't is your
fault. And yet people may tell you it is. If only you wouldn't
"flaunt" your sexuality, they might say. If you'd just kindly
refrain from "shoving it in people's faces," then people would
leave you alone. But that's crap, for two reasons:

1. Nothing you can do, short of physically harming
   someone else, justifies their physically harming you.
   If they hurt you, and you weren't hurting them first
   or credibly threatening to hurt them, they're the
   ones at fault. Period. Always.

2. When straight couples walk down the street holding hands or kiss in public, are they harassed or
   harmed for it? Not usually. Straight couples are free
   to "flaunt" their sexuality all day long, in public, on
   TV, everywhere. Saying you shouldn't have the same
   right just because you're not straight is hypocritical
   and unfair, and any behaviors that are fueled by that
   hypocrisy are the fault of the hypocrite, not you.

The same holds true for other couplings that are frowned
on by the Normalcy Police. Gray, a Black woman, gets it all
the time:

*I'll be walking down the street with a guy who's not Black
(someone I could very well just be friends with), and a
group of Black dudes will be like, "You know, you can
always come home," or, "I know he's not hittin' that, right?"
or tons of other stuff like that. It's really ridiculous—
especially when I think about how some of them had
dated white women.*

The bottom line is this: No one but you gets to say who
you love or who you're attracted to. And until we can create a
world where everyone actually behaves that way, the best thing
to do is get clear about that with yourself, so you can reject all
that misdirected blame that may come your way. (Well, that,
and get better at risk assessment, which we'll be getting into in
chapter 4.)

Rape

It's sick, but many people want to blame women for rape. Some
women blame it on the poor decisions other women make, because
they want to feel safe; they think if women get raped only when
they make "bad" choices—like walking alone at night, or going
home with a man they don't know very well—then they imagine they can avoid getting raped themselves by simply making
"smarter" decisions. Some guys blame women because they're
afraid to look at their own behaviors and attitudes, or they don't
want to believe that some dudes they know and like could be
violent criminals. Whatever their reasons, victim-blamers love to
point to women's sexuality as the reason they get raped.

And under this rationale, anything sexual can be called into question. Take these examples: When an eleven-year-old girl was gang-raped in Texas by eighteen young men, *The New York Times* focused on her behavior ("She dressed older than her age, wearing makeup and fashions more appropriate to a woman in her 20s. She would hang out with teenage boys at a playground, some said") and wondered how the perpetrators "could . . . have been drawn into such an act?"[5] And a judge in Manitoba refused to give a rapist who had told his victim the assault "would only hurt for a little while" any jail time, because she had "dressed in a tube top without a bra and jeans and [was] made up and wore high heels in a parking lot outside a bar, [making her] intentions publicly known that [she] wanted to party."[6]

And the list goes on . . . *Why were you wearing those heels/ that skirt/that dress if you didn't want it? Why were you dancing like that if you didn't want it? Why were you flirting with her if you didn't want it? Why did you kiss him if you didn't want to have sex with him? We know what you've done with other people, so you're obviously down for anything.* It's a familiar litany, but it's totally and completely bunk.

First of all, the logic doesn't hold up under scrutiny. Are these victim-blamers seriously saying that if you wear a pair of sexy shoes, then you're consenting to any and all sexual acts with anyone who might happen to see them? That's ridiculous, isn't it? But in addition to the fallacy of logic associated with blaming the victim, this line of argument is insulting to men, too. It assumes that men (the overwhelming majority of all rapists) are sexually incontinent—that if you turn them on they literally can't control themselves. Which is obviously untrue.

If it were true, most men *would* be rapists. Instead, researchers have found that only 4–8 percent of men are responsible for committing the vast majority of rapes.[7] Seems like most men are fully capable of flirting with a sexy woman and not committing a violent felony against her, doesn't it?

Also, the whole idea that women have to keep our sexuality in check so we don't get raped is an impossible trap. Are we supposed to never have fun? Never wear anything that makes us feel good? Are we supposed to police our own pleasure so that other people don't assault us? It's profoundly unfair and totally unrealistic. Even if you tried to do that, even if you believed it was your responsibility to never be sexual so that you'd never be raped, could you succeed? We all choose short-term pleasure over abstract risk some of the time. It's part of the human condition. And telling women we're not allowed to enjoy our bodies and our sexuality while men are allowed to do so freely is sexism of the highest order.

Finally, I'll repeat what I said earlier about homophobic attacks, because it applies here equally: Nothing you can do, short of physically harming someone else, justifies their physically harming you. If they hurt you, and you weren't hurting them first or credibly threatening to hurt them, they're the ones at fault. Period. Always.

Dive In: Think about times you've been blamed for something (nonsexual) that you knew wasn't your fault. List a few of them in your journal, then pick one and write about it. How did it feel to be blamed for

> something you didn't do? How did you maintain confidence in your innocence, despite other people's insistence you were guilty? Did you convince your accusers that you were not responsible? If so, how did you do that?

FEAR

It seems like there's so much to be afraid of when it comes to sex, doesn't it? Pregnancy, disease, violence, heartbreak, social rejection . . . I could go on and on. Fear is the number one tool folks use to try to control women's sexuality, and for good reason: It works. Why? Because some of these fears are based in reality. But a lot of them are exaggerated (like the risk of being attacked if you're walking around by yourself at night), and some of them are fabricated altogether (like the idea that having casual sex will make you incapable of bonding emotionally with a future partner), while some things that you might be afraid of if you knew about them—such as the many dangers that flow from not having direct, respectful communication with your sexual partners—don't get discussed at all. It's a mess, but it doesn't have to be.

All fears, whether real, imagined, or exaggerated, have one thing in common: The more energy you give them, the stronger they become. Am I saying that if you pretend STDs don't exist you'll never get one? Quite the opposite. If you're too afraid to talk about STDs, or learn about them, or negotiate safer sex with your partner, you're more likely to get infected. I used to teach self-defense to women, and one of the things I'd hear from many of my students was that they had been reluctant to take my class because thinking about having to use safety skills made them feel scared. Instead of dealing with that fear, instead of just feeling it and moving through it and moving on, they had been stuck, with fewer skills, and felt less safe as a result.

Let me put it another way: The best weapon against fear is information. You find yourself held back by fear? Investigate it. Ask yourself the following: How likely is it that this thing I fear will happen, really? How bad would it be if it happened? Is there anything I can do to make it less likely, or less awful if it happens? And: Where did I learn to be afraid of this? What might have motivated the people or institutions that taught me to be afraid? Do I feel good about those motives?

Let's practice by taking a deeper look at some of the most common fears women have about sex and sexuality.

Pregnancy

It's true that some kinds of sexual activity can put some of us at risk of becoming pregnant when we don't want to be. Fortunately, there's also a lot of good information about how to reduce and/or manage that risk.

A great place to start learning more about your birth control options is Planned Parenthood. You can visit their birth control info page online at www.wyrrw.com/ppbc, or, if there's a Planned Parenthood near you, make an appointment to go speak to one of their trained counselors, who can talk through your options and the risks with you and help you choose a method (or combination of methods) that feels right to you. If you can't get online or to a Planned Parenthood, another great resource is *Our Bodies, Ourselves,* which is all about women's health and has lots of good information about birth control options, risks, and effectiveness.

If you don't have access to any birth control, or none of those methods, even in combination, feel safe enough for you, there's plenty of sexual activity you can engage in that doesn't involve pregnancy risk. Masturbation, making out, all kinds of touching that don't involve a penis touching a vagina, oral sex, anal sex, mutual masturbation—take your pick. They're all incredibly low- or no-risk activities when it comes to pregnancy, and they can be lots and lots of fun.

Still worried? It may be time to ask yourself what you're really worried about and why. Some girls worry about pregnancy as a stand-in for the greater fear that engaging in sexuality will ruin their life. If that's the case for you, it's better to realize it sooner so that you can explore the real fear underneath and deal with it directly.

STDs

Sexually transmitted diseases (STDs) are serious. Some of them, like herpes, can't be cured, and if you get them, you'll have to deal with them for the rest of your life. Some of them, like HIV/AIDS, can kill you. Sometimes you can be infected and not know it at all, which puts you at risk of transmitting disease to other partners.

But STDs are also preventable. Yes, the old saying is true: The only truly safe sex is sex for one. But there are some basic ways to have partnered sexual interactions and keep the risk of transmitting disease very, very low. Get educated, decide how much risk is right for you, and you'll feel the fear melt away.

There are basically two approaches, which you can feel free to use in combination: barriers and behavior modification. Putting a latex barrier securely between you and the sexual fluids (and blood) of your partner significantly reduces the chance of catching a disease. And, if that's not enough for you, you can choose to engage only in sexual activities that don't bring you into contact with your partner's fluids.

Sound a lot like my advice on pregnancy prevention? That's because it is. And you should turn to the same resources to learn more: Planned Parenthood's page on STD prevention (www .wyrrw.com/ppss), a Planned Parenthood counselor, or *Our Bodies, Ourselves.*

And the same caveat holds true as well: If nothing quells your fears about STDs, it may be because this fear is a stand-in for deeper fears about sex. The sooner you can figure out what's really at the root of your fears, the sooner you'll be able to get what you really really want.

Rape

When we accept the blame for rape, even hypothetically, the fear of it can really hold us back. "I was taught 'sit with your legs closed. Don't be loud. Be damn near unnoticeable,'" says Gray, when she thinks about the rape-prevention messages her family taught her. "And now I feel like there's this constant corseting I do to myself. A conceptual corseting. It sounds terrible, but at one point, I was afraid of every man I saw on the street."

Gray is far from alone. One of the tricky parts of the pernicious myth that women bring rape on ourselves is that women internalize the blame and then start to worry that anything we do that's remotely sexual puts us in danger of being raped.

Let's clear this up now, shall we? You know what puts you in danger of being raped? Being in the presence of a rapist. You could be wearing seventy-three layers of shapeless, baggy sweats and still be raped if there's a rapist around. And you can wear your tightest, tiniest, hottest outfit and be completely safe if there's no one around who has the drive to violate you sexually. Thing is, the fear that acting sexy or sexual will get you raped is based on a misunderstanding of why and how rapists do the horrible things they do. Rapists don't attack because they want you so bad they can no longer control themselves. Rapists attack because they like raping. And the vast majority of them prefer raping victims they already know. They pick out their victims in advance and deliberately get them into situations where they're easy to attack. That means they don't look for victims who are super-sexy, they look for victims who they think will be easy to manipulate. That's why alcohol is so often involved with sexual assault: Rapists deliberately encourage their targets to get drunk so they'll be more malleable and less likely to fight back.

So go ahead. Wear what you like. Flirt how you like. Sleep with whom you want to. None of it is going to "get you" raped, because that's just not what rape is about.

And if you're still struggling with the fear of rape (after all, as many as one in five women in the United States will be raped in her lifetime; it's not an unreasonable thing to be afraid of), instead of curtailing your own activities, I strongly recommend taking some good self-defense training so you'll have some more tools with which to combat those fears. I'll talk more about self-defense in chapter 4.

Being Labeled a Slut or a Prude

Being called a slut or a prude hardly ever has anything to do with how much sex you are or aren't having. Girls who get labeled "sluts" are just girls who seem disobedient or threatening to the status quo. Sometimes this happens just because you have opinions and aren't afraid to speak up about them. Sometimes it happens because you've rejected blame and shame and that can seem like you're "out of control" to folks who haven't.

Girls who get labeled "prudes" aren't that different, actually. Maybe people call you a prude because you choose not to get drunk, or like to be sexual only with people you're in a committed relationship with. Sometimes it's just about your personal sense of style, or about someone else's cluelessness or mean agenda.

Twenty-three-year-old Prerna has felt this firsthand. "When I was upset with myself for sleeping with someone I didn't care about, my friend told me that I'm young and I 'should' be sleeping around without feeling bad about it," she recalls. "She thought she was releasing me from slut shame, but really she made me feel terrible about the fact that I want to be more selective with my sexual partners."

Don't let the fear of "getting a reputation" of any kind hold you back from exploring your sexuality on your own terms, even if that means you're not ready to explore it yet. Trust that you'll know when it's time.

At its core, the whole idea of the "slut" is based on an archaic double standard. Guys who sleep around gain status, but girls who do the same are seen as somehow damaged and suffering from low self-esteem. On the flip side, girls are often called "prudes" because they don't let peer pressure dictate how they experience sexuality. Guys who do the same thing are idolized as heroic. How you interact sexually is nobody's business but yours and your partner's, and as long as you're both having fun, being safe, and being respectful, it has no bearing on your value as a person.

No One Will Want Me

The fear of not being wanted is both powerful and seldom discussed. Many women are afraid to feel our own desire because we're afraid if we try to pursue it, we'll be rejected. And not just rejected by one particular person (after all, if you think you're pretty appealing, then one person's rejection won't matter that much). No, this fear is pervasive and personal, and there are any number of reasons why it might embed itself in your brain. For thirty-two-year-old Heidi, it went something like this: "Society has told me, day in and day out, that my body is too fat/too lumpy/too ugly/too unacceptable. That my body is too *much*. And I believed it because I didn't think I had any other option. According to this world, my body is wrong . . . and it's hard to imagine that anyone could possibly overlook that."

Maybe, like her, people have told you that you're undesirable, maybe even over and over. Maybe your body doesn't fit our narrow cultural beauty standard in one or more of an almost infinite number of ways. (We'll talk more about some of those ways in chapter 3.) Whatever the reason, there's only one thing you have to know: It's a lie.

No, I don't know you. I've never met you, never even seen a picture of you. But I can still promise you, right now, that you are desirable to someone. Probably lots of people.

Why? Because people are different and unpredictable. That's one of the awesome things about getting to know someone new: that moment when you find out she knows how to sword-fight, or he's an überfan of some obscure band you've never heard of before, but now that you're hearing them, you actually kind of love them—that crazy, quirky weirdness that makes us human also means that no two people have the exact same definition of "hot."

There are people in the world who will find the very qualities you hate about yourself—your skin, your butt, your laugh, whatever they are—completely irresistible. There are people in the world who will be incredibly turned on by other parts of your appearance you may not value as much as you should—like your strong shoulders, or the shape of your nose. And there are people in the world who just don't care very much about appearance, period. They're going to be attracted to you because of who you are and how you act.

The flip side of this is the fear of being wanted for the "wrong reasons," which goes a little like this: The only people who want me don't want me at all, but want something that I symbolize to them. This can be a pretty painful experience for lots of women, including women of color, fat women, trans or genderqueer women, etc., who are often treated as fetish objects instead of as whole people. (We'll get further into navigating "wrong reasons" land mines in chapter 6.)

Ultimately, living in fear of rejection can make it much harder to discover and articulate what you really really want. As Phoebe, forty-four, puts it, "I know my vulnerability is around not feeling attractive. But what that fear leads me to is a bigger one: that I'll lose the ability to even know what I want in a sexual situation, because I'll be trying to read what the other person wants. And that fear is paralyzing to me."

Put another way: The energy you spend denying your desires for fear of rejection is energy spent sabotaging the chance you'll see those desires fulfilled. On the other hand, the more energy you spend making friends with what you want, the better your chances of getting the opportunity to fulfill those desires.

I Want the Wrong Things

There are all kinds of desires that can feel "wrong." Depending on your background, it can feel "wrong" to want to be sexual with women or transgender people. It can feel wrong to want to act on certain fantasies. It can feel wrong to want to be sexual at all. If you're feeling confused about what's wrong and what isn't, the best person to ask is *you:* Go reread your sexual mission statement.

But sometimes we want things that may actually be wrong. Maybe we want someone who's in a monogamous partnership with someone else. Maybe we want someone who doesn't want us, and we want to force them to be sexual with us. Maybe we want someone who is off-limits because the power differential is too dangerous: a boss or a student or a friend's parent.

It's important to know that we all want "wrong" things at one point or another. Our culture's standard of what's acceptable sexual behavior for women is so narrow it's impossible to live up to. So if you find yourself fearing your own desires because you think they're "wrong," the best thing to do is take the time to figure out which kind of "wrong" they are. Specifically, you want to ask yourself: If I acted on this desire, would anyone get hurt? If so, who and why?

Sometimes this feeling of "wrong" stems from a desire we just can't let ourselves articulate to ourselves. In her book *Dilemmas of Desire,* researcher Deborah Tolman talked with many teenage girls who'd experienced this phenomenon. One girl in particular, fifteen-year-old Megan, told Tolman about her struggles acknowledging her same-sex attractions:

There was this one girl that I had kinda liked from school . . . we were sitting next to each other during the movie and, kind of her leg was on my leg and I was like, wow, you know . . . But it's so impossible, I think I just like block it out, I mean, it could never happen . . . I just can't know what I'm feeling.[8]

Later, Megan tells Tolman more explicitly: "You know it's like scary . . . it's society . . . you never would think of, you know, it's natural to kiss a girl."

Even if you do find yourself wanting something you think would hurt yourself or someone else, I should stress here that there are no wrong *desires,* only some wrong *actions.* It's very common to fantasize about things you would never actually do in real life, and there's nothing bad about that. We'll talk more about that kind of desire in chapter 8.

> **Dive In:** Make a list of things that scare you about sex. Don't worry if those fears seem rational to you or not—just write them all down. Now circle the three that scare you the most. Of those three, pick one, and write for five minutes about why that thing scares you and how bad it would be if that scary thing happened. Then reread what you've just written, and write for five more minutes taking the other position: arguing why that feared thing is unlikely to happen, or easily preventable, or not that bad after all.

Sensing a theme here? The Terrible Trio can be powerful and insidious, but you don't have to let them rule you. And your best defense against them is information: separating fact from fiction, yes, but also separating the things you've been taught to believe about sex from what actually makes sense to you when you really think about it. Ever heard the phrase "sunlight is the best disinfectant"? It applies here, and what it means is this: If you're infected with the Terrible Trio, the best way to get rid of them is to shine the light of fact and thought on them.

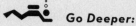 **Go Deeper:**

1. Take a big blank page in your journal and write your name in the very center. Then think about the people who've influenced the way you feel about your sexuality and yourself. Put the names of those who've influenced you most closest to you, and the ones who've influenced you less farther away, to make a cluster diagram. Now mark the ones who encourage you to feel shame, blame, or fear about your sexuality with an "S," "B," or "F," as appropriate. And mark the ones who encourage you to reject the Terrible Trio with a star. Now make a new diagram. This time, put the people you want to have the most influence on you closest to you, and those whose influence you want to minimize farthest away.

2. Using magazines or the Internet, find images that represent all the bad things you can think of that are blamed on sexual women. Make a collage of these images, print it out if it's online, and then take the collage, a deep metal bowl, and some matches over to a sink or bathtub. Making sure that nothing flammable is nearby, put the collage in the bowl and the bowl in the sink or bathtub, and then light it on fire and watch it burn. (Alternative: If burning isn't practical where you live, run it through a shredder, soak it in water until it disintegrates, or rip it into tiny pieces.)

3. Make a list of names used for prudes and sluts. Write another list of names—at least as long as the first one—for women who are proud and sexual. Make these up if you need to.

4. Write a list of five sexual practices that are con-
    sidered taboo. Write a list of five sexual things
    you enjoy doing.

5. Write a letter to someone who put you down,
    letting them know how hurtful this felt (an ex, an
    advertiser, a boss, a friend).

6. Write a letter to someone telling them how much
    you value how they see you and understand who
    you really are.

CHAPTER 3

I'M OKAY,
YOU'RE OKAY

S O, NOW THAT YOU'VE FINISHED CHAPTERS 1 AND 2, YOU'VE
sorted out your own beliefs from the forces that have influenced you and rejected the Terrible Trio. You're all set, right?

Just kidding. Of course you're not! This is a long journey,
and you're off to a good start. But a word of patience: Change
doesn't happen overnight, and it doesn't happen all in a neat
little line, either. You may have epiphanies along the way that
make you feel clearer than you've ever been, and then the next
day something can happen—someone says something to you,
you see something on TV, maybe it's something in this book—
that throws you for a loop, and you feel more confused than
ever. That's normal. You're in the process of reevaluating a
pretty deeply rooted part of your identity. It's going to be a
bumpy ride for at least part of it. So, if you're feeling great right
now and can't wait to dive in further, that's awesome. And if
you're feeling overwhelmed or confused, that's okay, too. It just
means you're on the journey, and that's what counts. Just keep

doing your daily writing and your weekly body love, and keep coming back to these exercises. We'll get there together.

In this chapter, we're going to go a little deeper into some of the forces that may have shaped the way you think about your own sexuality, and others' as well. Specifically, we're going to explore group identities and the sexual assumptions that are attached to them. And then we're going to see if we might want to detach 'em a little.

It's useful, too, to think about these issues not just in terms of how they affect you, but also in terms of how they might affect a current or future sexual partner. Not just because it will make you a better lover and friend, but because it's sometimes easier to start by empathizing with a loved one, and then extend that same kind of empathy to ourselves. But before we do this, a reminder: There's no way to ever be fully free of the lessons we've learned at a deep level about sex, and that holds for the messages that come with your identities, too. You may embrace or even embody some of the stereotypes that are unfairly applied to you, and that's fine. Even if you act the exact opposite of how you're expected to, you're still behaving in some ways in response to how you've been taught to act. And the social forces that keep these stereotypes in place are strong—as much as we wish it could be, it's not possible to just erase them. The goal here isn't to wipe your slate clean, it's to take a look at the ingredients that have brought you to where you are with your sexuality today and adjust the seasonings until you think you're delicious.

AGE

Age is unlike most other group identities in that it's always fundamentally changing for everyone. And yet your age can have a lot to do with how you feel about your sexuality, how other people view your sexuality, and how you view others' sexuality.

Let's take the most obvious example: Most young women are expected to be innocent virgins. That's not redundant, because just being a virgin isn't enough to live up to social expectations. To avoid judgment, young women shouldn't even be curious about or desirous of sex. Nowhere is this more apparent than in the ongoing debate about whether or not insurance companies should cover a vaccine for HPV (human papillomavirus), an STD that sometimes causes cervical cancer. The vaccine is quite effective when given to girls before they become sexually active, and that's just what gets some folks upset: They fear that even talking about STD prevention in the process of giving a girl a shot will turn her into a sex-crazed maniac. They'd prefer that girls grow up with a greater risk of dying from cervical cancer than to suggest in any way that it might be okay for girls to have a thought related to sex.[1]

The folks who push the message that girls shouldn't be thinking about sex say it's about teaching girls to value themselves, but if they'd rather girls die of cancer than be sexual, that doesn't really value girls much, does it? What it really teaches is that the most important part of a girl's character is what she does or doesn't want to do with her body—not how good a friend she is, how hard she works in school, how honest she is, or anything else.

What does this mean for you? Well, for one thing, if you're a young woman, it means extra pressure to not even *think* about being sexual. It means that if you do think about or act on your sexuality in any way, you may feel afraid to talk with anyone about it, which is isolating and can be dangerous.

In fact, the pressure on younger women to be "good" (that is, not sexual) can be so great that it isolates us not only from older adults, but also from other young women. Eugenia, seventeen, had promised to tell her best friend when she had sex with her boyfriend for the first time. "But then, when it happened, I didn't think I wanted to," she told Deborah Tolman, "and it wasn't like I myself felt bad about it, but I just didn't want to, 'cause I felt good about it, and I didn't want anyone else passing judgment on me, that's what it was."[2]

On the flip side of that coin, young women are also treated as the most desirable sex objects there are and are pressured to act as sexy as possible—wear sexy Halloween costumes, work out to stripper-pole aerobics, and wear panties that say WHO NEEDS CREDIT CARDS . . . [3] These sexual expressions aren't about the girls engaging in them, they're about fulfilling the fantasies of heterosexual men. So, to review what's expected of you if you're a young woman in our culture: Be drop-dead sexy, but don't think about sex ever. Good luck with that.

And, because women get shamed coming and going, older women face certain assumptions and stigmas as well. Past a certain, nebulous (though still fairly young) age, women are considered prudish or frigid if they're not sexually desirous and experienced. And that kind of pressure can be just as isolating if it doesn't match up with how you actually feel.

Or, if older women are sexually desirous and experienced and happen to have a partner who's younger than they are, they're called "cougars" or "pumas" or some other predatory-cat name, and become the butt of jokes.

Or, if older women start looking like, well, older women—as they naturally will—we suddenly assume that they've lost any sexual drive they may have once had, or, worse, any sexual desirability. Furthermore, younger women sometimes assume that their foremothers are easily scandalized by the sexual antics of young women. This is too bad for many reasons, not the least of which is that some older women have been through a lot of what young women are just starting to experience and can share their wisdom about how to navigate the tricky waters of sexuality, if only young women would ask.

Are you noticing what I am? There's basically no right age to be in this paradigm. You'll always be accused of being too young or too old to behave or think or feel a certain way. And whatever age you are, there are only wrong ways to be sexual. Know what that means? The whole paradigm is a trap.

Dive In: Imagine you're twenty years older or younger than you are now. Think about what life might be like for you then, sexually speaking. What did/will people expect you to act like, and what do you think you might want or have wanted to be doing sexually? Now take on the voice of that older or younger self, and write your current-day self a letter. What would your future or past self want your present self to know about sex and sexuality?

RACE

As with all things racial, the intersection of race and sexuality is complicated. It's complicated by the ways race and economic class intersect, by the history of slavery in the United States and around the world, by the fact that race is both an utterly bogus way to look at people and simultaneously very real. And yet while it's definitely not simple, it sure is important to think about.

Consider, for example, the "innocent virgin" we were describing in the section on age earlier in this chapter. Picture her in your mind's eye. Maybe take a moment now to draw a picture of her, or write down a description of what she looks like.

What did you draw or describe? Was it a white girl with long hair? Maybe blond, blue-eyed, or freckle-faced?

If it was, it's not an accident. Because we live in a racist society that values white girls more than girls of color, we tend to imagine that purity is pale. That assumption has a terrible flip side: Girls of color are often viewed as always sexually available, simply because of their race. Just look at the specific stereotypes: Latina women are "spicy," Middle Eastern and South Asian women are simultaneously "exotic" and "repressed," Asian women are "submissive," Black women are "wild" or "animalistic"—it doesn't matter what disgusting stereotype you choose; it boils down to the same thing: Women of color are assumed to be always available for sex.

"It's easy to feel cheap when you have dark skin, frizzy hair, and a big butt," says Mag. "TV, magazines, people on the street, people in class—it seems like everyone feels like they have a need, no, a right, to your body that you don't have. I've had random white children come up to me and slap my ass. I've had men take photos while I wasn't looking, or strangers come up to me and 'compliment' me on how luscious my backside looks, and what they'd like to do with me."

You're smart enough to see how ridiculous assumptions about the sexualities of women of color are. Of course every individual woman wants different things that have nothing to do with her skin color. But the problem with this paradigm goes past how reductive it is. By treating women as though their race dictates their sexuality, we're also telling women that their actual desires don't matter and probably shouldn't even exist. As you know by now, nothing could be further from the truth.

But it gets even more twisted: Because of these racial stereotypes, many girls of color are pressured by their families and communities to live the stereotypes down by (sing it with me if you know the tune by now) being unimpeachably innocent of sexual desire. So the wider culture is sexualizing girls of color right and left, and yet, in the end, they still often get shoved into the same virginity trap as do white girls.

On top of all of this, it's important to keep in mind one of the main reasons women of color are expected to be always sexually available—because in countries where they've been historically enslaved or colonized by white cultures, the white men in those cultures felt free to rape them with impunity. That women of color in colonized countries should have any say-so in what happens to their bodies, sexually or otherwise, is a pretty new idea in the grand scheme of things, and one that women of color have had to fight hard for, and still have to fight for today.

For some women of color in colonized countries, getting in touch with their ancestors' pre-colonization attitudes toward sexuality can be profoundly healing or liberating. Jessica Yee, founder of the Native Youth Sexual Health Network, explains it this way: "As I have listened to my grandmothers explain to me, sex used to be sacred and even upheld as an enjoyable part of our life as First Nations people. . . . Colonization, Christianization, and genocidal oppression have drastically severed the ties to traditional knowledge that would enable us to make informed choices about our sexual health and relationships. The fact is that many of our communities are reluctant to go anywhere near the topic of sexual health because it is viewed as 'dirty,' 'wrong,' or a 'White man's thing.' We carry a long history of being sexually exploited, from the early Pocahontas and squaw days right up to the modern oversexualization of 'easy' Native women that permeates so much of the media. . . . In generic sexual health campaigns, I often hear the slogan 'Respect Yourself, Protect Yourself'—which I have always found to be incomplete. In our communities, I say, 'Respect Yourself, Protect Yourself, and Be Proud of Your Culture'—because that last element will enable us to accomplish the first two."

> **Dive In:** Obviously, there's a heck of a lot to work through when it comes to unpacking the sexual suitcase your racial identity comes with. Before you can get into it, though, you need an answer to this question:

What is your racial identity? Notice I didn't say "you need *the* answer to this question." Your answer can be anything that makes sense to you. It can be a word, a sentence, or a paragraph. Whatever it is, give it some thought, and then take a minute to write it down.

Now, write a list of sexual stereotypes that are associated with your racial identity in the community or country you're currently living in (or the community or country you were raised in, if that's a more useful point of reference). Then take or draw a picture of yourself and put it in the middle of a big piece of paper. Next, write each of those stereotypes in a cloud around your picture, with the ones that are closest to true about you nearest to you, and the ones that are the least true for you farthest away. It's okay if some stereotypes apply to you, or if none of them do. What matters is that you're at the center of your identity, not the stereotypes.

CLASS

Economic class can be difficult to talk about. It's about more than just how much money you or your family make or have made at any given moment. It also has to do with how much money you had growing up, what kind of education you had access to, your parents' class backgrounds, and how you were taught to think about money and class.

When it comes to sexuality, class functions a lot like race. Girls from lower-class families are stereotyped as "fast." Middle-class girls are expected to be "good." And upper-class girls—think Paris Hilton or the Kardashians—can pretty much do whatever they want. And the same pressure is applied to the marginalized girls, the ones thought of as always available, to live down those stereotypes by being extra pure.

It gets even more complicated in the place where economic pressures interact directly with sex. I'm talking about sex work, of course, which includes all jobs in which people exchange sexual services or performances for money. That could be anything from prostitution to stripping to acting in porn films to being a waitress in a sexualized establishment like Hooters.

Most of the people doing sex work are women, and just as there's a wide variety of sex work that women do, there is also a real range of reasons why women do sex work. Some women and girls have no choice; they're victims of what's called "sexual trafficking," which means they're basically kidnapped and forced to do sex work. Some women, however, have lots of choices and choose to do sex work because they find it enjoyable and rewarding. The majority of sex workers fall somewhere in between: They haven't been kidnapped, but they don't have a lot of good choices available to them, either. Maybe they haven't had access to education or skills training, or maybe they live somewhere where the economy is poor and no one is hiring. It's also true that women across the board are paid less than men for the same work: about 70 cents for every dollar a man gets paid. Often, sex work pays better than most other jobs women have a chance of getting. So what's the point? That many women who choose sex work (as opposed to being trafficked into it) choose it for largely economic reasons.

Beyond sex work, women are constantly exposed to more mundane sex-money interactions. Consider them the big sisters to the old if-a-guy-pays-for-dinner-you-owe-him-sex trope.

Bartending and waiting tables, people assume that because you work in a serving profession, you're open for business. That if they tip you well, you might go home with them. {Shana}

For example, consider the woman who has to choose between leaving a partner who's not healthy to be with and having a place to live for herself and/or her kids. This happens all the time. If she breaks up with her partner, she loses her partner's financial support, which is all that's between her and a pretty dire situation. Or what about a woman who is trying to get ahead in her career in order to create a better economic situation for herself, only to be forced to deal with the sexual attention of a boss or colleague? That's a big reason sexual harassment laws exist—so that women don't have to choose between economic freedom and sexual freedom. But it can be hard to prove harassment, and there's a lot of pressure on women in male-dominated workplaces to "be able to take a compliment," "be one of the boys," or comply with other "boys will be boys" codes that ultimately mean that women who call out powerful men in the workplace about their harassing behavior can expect to be punished—even fired—instead of being helped.

Women's sexuality is also often policed on the job: Women are vulnerable to criticism and punishment from higher-ups if they're deemed "too sexy" or "not sexy enough" for the workplace. We're still far from a day when women are truly free of sexual pressure on the job.

Reproductive freedom is also influenced by economics and class. If you can afford birth control and STD prevention and testing, or have access to insurance that covers it, you're going to be able to manage the risks that come with sex a lot better than if you don't have that kind of access. The same goes for access to abortion. In the United States, it's illegal for any federal money to pay for abortion, and that means that people who rely on Medicaid or other federal programs for their healthcare have no practical access to abortion.

My family is quite wealthy, so I have enough disposable income to buy really high-quality safer-sex equipment, and sex equipment in general. And that affects the way that I've been able to be sexual. {Enoch, age nineteen}

Dive In: Think about a time when your sexual expressions or actions have been influenced by your class or economic situation. Write about that time for five minutes. Now imagine your situation had been different—maybe you had more or less money, or a different class background. How would your choices have been different in that situation? Write about that alternative reality for five more minutes.

GENDER

It may seem strange to have a section about how gender affects sexuality in a book that's explicitly for women, because in many ways, this whole book is about how gender affects sexuality. But gender isn't just a question with two answers, one for women and one for men.

What do I mean by this, exactly? A few different things. For one, women are often stereotyped into gender categories depending on their behavior. For example, women who are loud, ambitious, opinionated, or aggressive are often considered "unfeminine," no matter what they look like or how they carry themselves. And women express gender in all kinds of different ways. Some women are incredibly "girlie"—they like pink and lace and makeup and delicate, shiny things. Some women are androgynous, which means that they're neither masculine nor feminine, or else that they're fairly equal parts of both. Some women are straight-up masculine, preferring short haircuts, work boots or sneakers to heels, and men's shirts to women's blouses. (I'm being a little reductive here, as gender expression is about much more than what you wear or how you groom yourself, but I'm using these visual examples as a kind of shorthand to get to my larger point.)

Women also vary in gender in ways that go deeper than gender expression. Some of us identify as "genderqueer," a term that means different things to different people, but that generally means that the person using it doesn't feel like their gender can be described by the gender binary (the idea that there are only two genders, "man" and "woman"). Some women identify as women even though they were born as biological males. And many trans women do not identify as having ever been biologically male. These women usually call themselves transgender. Then there are women who were born with ambiguous genitals and the doctors decided they should be raised as women (often these women had involuntary surgery, as babies, to remove the "nonfemale" parts of their bodies). These women often identify as intersex.

Why bother describing all of these gender differences if we're all women? You can probably guess the answer: because gender expression and identity are used all the time to limit women's sexual choices. We assume that masculine women want to have sex only with other women, when many of them like sex with men. We treat transgender and intersex women like freaks who are only allowed to have a sexuality if they're willing to be objects of fascination to fetishize, and whose genuine sexual desire is treated as disgusting and dangerous. We assume that very feminine women are pure and passive and malleable (and heterosexual, of course!), just waiting for a strong man to come along and marry them.

It's also true that women who are gender "transgressive" in any way are often assumed to be either sexually untouchable or hypersexual. Enoch says:

When I became really visibly queer, all of a sudden everyone I knew thought I was having a ton of sex. At the time I was still horrified by the idea of sex and I had all of these really huge boundaries and was really inaccessible sexually, but everybody thought I was having all this sex. And

*it was really confusing to me, because the assumption
that was made was, Oh, you know what your sexuality is,
so you're doing things with it. But I really, really wasn't.*

You can also probably guess by now that none of these stereotypes reflect the wide range of sexualities experienced by the
women in these groups. And you can further guess that now's
an awfully good time to take a look at the nuances of your own
gender expression and identity, and the baggage that may come
along with them.

> **Dive In:** Using magazines and the Internet,
> collect images of people whose gender expression seems
> similar to yours. Then take a look at them all together:
> What do the images have in common? What words could
> be used to describe these people? Write down at least
> ten words.

SEXUAL ORIENTATION

It may seem overobvious to say that sexual orientation inter-
acts with sexual identity, but the interactions can and do go far
beyond simply the gender of your preferred partners.

Let's start at the beginning. Everyone has a sexual orientation. All that means is that you're attracted to some particular
combination of genders or gender expressions. The most well-
known terms for sexual orientation are "straight" or "gay," but
that's far from a complete list. Some people identify as bisexual,

which means they're attracted to both men and women. Some people are attracted only to masculinity or femininity, regardless of gender. And there are endless combinations. Personally, I identify as "flexisexual," a word I invented because I'm attracted to more than just men and women, and because my patterns of attraction have changed over time. Some people do find that their sexual orientation changes throughout their lifetime, while others consider it a completely fixed part of their identity. There's no right or wrong answer, but it's worth thinking about: What's your sexual orientation?

Whatever your answer, it can have an impact on what people expect from you sexually, and therefore what you expect from yourself. What's more, it can also affect how comfortable you feel discussing and exploring your sexuality, which can have a major impact on your ability to know what you really really want.

This impact is most obvious for women who identify as lesbian, bi, or queer or have other nonheterosexual identities. Queer women are still treated by many people as "sick" or "unnatural." Nothing could be further from the truth, of course. No one sexual orientation is more or less natural than any other, including heterosexuality, but the pervasive belief that straight is "right" can lead queer-identified women to try to deny their sexual orientation to themselves or others, feel shame, or otherwise cut themselves off from their sexuality.

Dive In: Make a list of all the words you can think of that you've used yourself or heard someone else use to describe someone's sexual orientation. Don't hold back—list the slang and slur words right alongside the more formal terms. Next, cross out every word that you think no one should ever use about anyone. Then cross out every word that you personally would never use to describe someone else. Then, of the remaining words, cross out every one that you wouldn't want anyone else to use when describing you. Lastly, cross out any word that's left that you would never use to describe yourself.

Write all of the words that are left in a new list. How do they make you feel? Do they describe your sexual orientation? Are there facets of your orientation that words don't exist for? If you feel like it, invent a word that helps fill in those gaps.

BODY TYPE

Do you feel complicated emotions around your body when it comes to sex? You're not alone. A 2011 survey of British women found that 52 percent of them avoid sex because they feel bad about how their bodies look, 13 percent have sex only in the dark because they don't want to be seen naked, and 10 percent avoid sexual positions they'd otherwise enjoy because they feel ashamed about various parts of their bodies.[4]

We rely on body shape and size far too much when deciding who's sexy and who's sexual. Women who are flat-chested and not very curvy are often assumed to be asexual or docile or attracted to women, while women with fuller breasts and some curve to their hips are assumed to be always-ready, indiscriminate sex machines. (These body types map somewhat to racial stereotypes, too: The "hot-blooded" Latina is likely to be curvier than the "ready-to-serve" Asian.)

Because our culture has a super-narrow definition of what kind of female body is sexy, most women feel insecure about theirs. There are all kinds of things a body can do or be that will land it outside the "sexy" box. You could be short. You could have blemishes on your skin. You could have short or coarse or frizzy or thinning hair. The more ways your body goes against the "sexy" standard, the less desirable you're assumed to be.

Another example of ways in which your body might not fit into the social standard of sexy is if you're fat. (It's okay to say "fat": Fat people tend to know they're fat. It's a descriptive word. It doesn't have to be a slur unless you mean it that way.) Fat women are treated as utterly undesirable in our culture. Similar to the ways transgender and intersex women are treated, when it comes to sex, fat women are often turned into a "bizarre" fetish object. The result is that fat women are told to be grateful for any sexual attention they receive from anyone, whether they themselves find that person sexually appealing or not. In other words, even more than your average women, fat women are only allowed to be occasional objects of desire and are regularly denied their right to have and pursue sexual desires of their own.

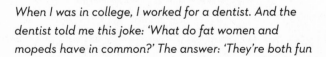

When I was in college, I worked for a dentist. And the dentist told me this joke: 'What do fat women and mopeds have in common?' The answer: 'They're both fun

to ride, but you wouldn't want to be seen with them in public.' And it felt horrible to hear, but then part of me was like, What do you mean, they'd be fun to ride? I felt it was just so clear that you don't get to play in this arena because you're large. {Phoebe, age forty-four}

This way of thinking becomes very dangerous when sexual violence is mixed in. When fat women are raped, they're often told they should be grateful that anyone wanted them, or, alternatively, disbelieved because it doesn't seem plausible that anyone would want them "enough to rape them." These arguments not only rely on the dangerous myth that rape is about uncontrollable sexual desire (it's *not*), but also propagate the message that fat women's bodies aren't valuable enough to the culture for their violation to be taken seriously. (For more resources on body acceptance, I highly recommend Kate Harding and Marianne Kirby's book *Lessons from the Fat-o-sphere.*)

Another variety of experience is when your body is disabled or in some way functions differently than most people expect it to. If your physical difference is easy to spot visually, because you walk with a cane, or use a wheelchair, or have a prosthetic limb, you'll likely be subjected to many of the same treatments that fat people get. Plus, you'll have the added "bonus" of many people's assuming you're not even physically capable of having sex or sexual desire.

But some less visible physical differences can also have a big impact on the room the culture makes for your sexuality. For example, there is no sign for "consent" in sign language. The concept of sexual consent literally doesn't exist in the language many deaf people use to communicate. When you combine that glaring absence with the poor or nonexistent education and social services many deaf people have access to, it creates obstacles to their ability to conceive of and express their sexuality that many hearing people can scarcely imagine.

What's extra sad about all of these social limitations put on women with "nonideal" bodies is that, in reality, there are people who have genuine sexual desires for all different kinds of women's bodies. It's probably true that conventionally pretty women get more sexual attention than women whose bodies fall significantly outside the norm, because we all get trained about what we "should" find attractive, and people who sleep with women aren't immune to that socialization. There are social consequences for people who are attracted to "nonideal" women, too, and many folks don't want to pay that price, or have never considered that they could opt out of the limited system they were handed. But there are also people of all genders who have spent some time figuring out what they really really want, and those people have an infinite variety of sexual appetites. After all, the women in that British study I referenced are the ones avoiding sex, having it with the lights out, and limiting their own sexual positions. Know what that means? They have willing sex partners who want them. It's the women themselves who are holding themselves back based on their fears about their own bodies.

What's more, healthy sexual partners will be attracted by your confidence and comfort in your own skin, sometimes even more than by the details of your physical body. Feminist theorist bell hooks learned this lesson personally. In her book

Communion: The Female Search for Love, she recalls that "when I was thin anorexically and had difficulty eating, I had far fewer partners than during years when I chose to be healthy and to affirm and admire that as the most vital sign of beauty."[5] And she challenges us all to do the same:

Grown women raised to hate their bodies can change their minds . . . They can begin to do the work of becoming self-loving by first reclaiming the right to inhabit a healthy body and to identify that as the foundation of beauty and attractiveness. This is one of those cultural revolutions that can take place just by our saying no. . . . Saying no to any devaluation and debasement of the female body is a loving practice.

Dive In: List your five favorite body parts, and pay them outrageous compliments. Go wild! Use your name. ("Jaclyn. You have the cutest knees! I love the way they are round and dimpled! Your knees work so hard every day!")

SEXUAL TRAUMA

If you've already been the victim of a sexual trauma (such as incest, molestation, or sexual assault), first of all, I'm very sorry. It happened to me, too, and I know there's nothing I can say to make the pain of it go away. I also know that there's nothing shameful about it—whatever happened, you didn't do anything shameful in that situation. The person who violated you did.

There's no "right answer" when considering the ways sexual trauma might impact your sexuality. Many survivors of sexual violence suffer from post-traumatic stress disorder (PTSD), and PTSD can lead to disassociation, an increase in risk-taking behaviors, and increased risk of addiction—all symptoms that can complicate a survivor's relationship to sex. So it's no surprise that some survivors find that sex—or certain kinds of it—becomes very difficult for them, because it reminds them too much of the assault. Others develop unhealthy sexual compulsions that expose them to unnecessary emotional and physical risks.

Unfortunately, many people generalize this possibility of sexual dysfunction into a belief that women who've experienced sexual trauma are sexually "damaged," and attribute any kind of sexual behavior on our part to our trauma. The problem with applying this stereotype to any particular survivor is that none of us can be reduced to a statistic. Knowing something is more or less likely about a group we belong to doesn't actually tell you anything about us in particular. If I told you that women with brown eyes are more likely to have brown hair, and you know I have brown eyes, could you know that my hair is brown? Of course not. And assuming an abuse survivor has an unhealthy relationship with sex is equally wrong. What's more, it yet again takes control away from the survivor when it comes to what she does or doesn't want to do with her body. Melissa McEwan, writing at her blog, Shakesville, tells of the terrible impact this dynamic had on her after she was raped:

I'd spent my life learning that my worth as a female person was attached to my virginity. My value as an unsullied cunt was gone; I tried instead to find value as a girl who knew how to give great head.

And, you know, that almost worked for a while.

There exists a stereotype, a myth, that sexual trauma makes women more promiscuous. (And some women do react to sexual violence with promiscuity; there is no one singular, textbook, universal response to rape, no "right way" to be a survivor.) But it wasn't rape that made me more promiscuous than I otherwise might have been; it was the idea that I had lost my worth as a human and some fundamental goodness which had been wrapped inside my virginity.[6]

Women who've experienced sexual trauma should be just as free as women who haven't to have sex (or not) on our own terms. Some of us may choose to stop having sex for a while, while others may find that having consensual sex helps us regain a feeling of control over our sexual choices. Many of us will find that one approach works for a while, then something shifts and another approach seems more appealing. The most healing thing I've found is to find a way to feel in control of your sexual choices. Which is how everyone should feel!

In other words, what matters isn't that we conform to some idea of how abuse victims are supposed to behave, but rather, that whatever sex we're having feels healthy and supportive to us and our partners. And that's not something that anyone else gets to decide for you.

> ≈≋ **Dive In:** Write a list of groups you belong to that there are stereotypes about (racial/ethnic groups, people who participate in a particular hobby or interest you have, people who share your body type or sexual orientation, etc.) and then write down the most common stereotypes people have about each of those groups. When you're done, circle all the stereotypes that are actually true of you, and put an "x" through the ones that don't apply. Now, spend five minutes writing about how it feels when someone uses a stereotype to assume something about you that turns out to be true, and another five minutes writing about when someone stereotypes you in a way that isn't true at all.

STEREOTYPING OTHERS

So far, we've focused pretty exclusively on how stereotyping can make it harder for you to figure out and pursue what you really really want. But stereotyping cuts both ways. Just as we're all taught to believe certain things about sexuality long before we can decide for ourselves what makes sense, none of us are immune to stereotypes about others. In a practical sense, that means that each of us is constantly making assumptions about other people based on limited information. You see an older woman and assume she'd be scandalized if she knew what you did last night. You see a masculine-looking woman and assume she is attracted to women and likes to open doors. You see a dark-skinned woman and assume she's "exotic" and "easy." You see a fat woman and assume she has no sexuality whatsoever.

Of course, you—you personally, you, sitting right there reading this—may not make any or all of these assumptions, but I guarantee you make some of your own. On the one hand, that's okay, in the sense that it's unavoidable. No one is ever completely free from stereotypes. It's just as impossible as becoming completely free of all the forces that influenced how you experience sexuality. But just like with those forces, the more you become aware of the stereotypes you do hold, the easier it becomes to minimize them and the damage they can do.

And yes, I said "damage." Stereotyping other people is always damaging. Who gets damaged and how depends on how you act out your bias. If you make a comment to a friend about another girl's "slutty" clothing, you're damaging both the friend (by being yet another force that's telling her that there's a "right" and "wrong" way to express her sexuality through dress) and possibly the person you're commenting on (if your comments and the shaming they contain find their way back to her ears). If you treat a woman in a wheelchair as though she's a child and has no sexuality, or if you act shocked when she expresses her sexuality somehow, you're definitely damaging her by reinforcing artificial limitations on her sexuality that, I promise you, she had to work hard to overcome in order to express her sexuality in the first place.

But what if you don't express your stereotypes out loud? What if you just think them to yourself? That's better than acting on them, to be sure. But you may still be conveying your assumptions through subconscious behaviors. And even if you're not, even if you just see someone on the street and stereotype them in your mind as they walk by without even noticing you, well, you're still doing damage. You're doing damage to yourself. You're sending your own self a message, which is that it's totally fair to make assumptions about someone's sexuality based on no real information. And that hurts you in two ways: (1) It cuts you off from learning about the real experiences and perspectives of people who may differ from you, which may mean you never connect with someone who could be a great friend or lover, or just that you lack some crucial information about the world, and (2) it sends you a message: Stereotypes are true. And that makes it harder for you to reject the stereotypes that others try to put on you.

> ≋ **Dive In:** For the next week, see how many times you can catch yourself thinking or acting based on stereotypes. Don't judge—we all do it. Just observe yourself, and keep a log of each example you can catch.

Feeling frustrated by all of these social forces trying to limit your sexual options? You're not alone. Don't take it out on yourself—do something about it. When you find yourself butting up against oppressive stereotypes (or worse), try to channel your feelings outward, into outrage or action, as opposed to turning inward with feelings of hopelessness or inadequacy. Don't worry if you're not perfect at this—it takes a lot of practice. We'll talk in more detail in chapter 6 about dealing with difficult emotions, and in chapter 11 about ways to get involved with changing the sexual culture for everyone. And if you're interested in exploring any of the issues raised in this chapter in more depth, and connecting with other people working on them, definitely check out www.wyrrw.com/ch3resources, as well as the following books:

- *Sex Ed and Youth: Colonization, Sexuality and Communities of Colour,* edited by Jessica Yee
- *Black Sexual Politics: African Americans, Gender, and the New Racism,* by Patricia Hill Collins
- *Lessons from the Fat-o-sphere: Quit Dieting and Declare a Truce with Your Body,* by Kate Harding and Marianne Kirby
- *Exile and Pride: Disability, Queerness and Liberation,* by Eli Clare
- *Gender Outlaws: The Next Generation,* edited by Kate Bornstein and S. Bear Bergman
- *Persistence: All Ways Butch and Femme,* edited by Ivan Coyote and Zena Sharman
- *Outdated: Why Dating Is Ruining Your Love Life,* by Samhita Mukhopadhyay

(And other fab books listed at www.wyrrw.com/ch3 resources!)

 Go Deeper:

1. Take out the timeline you started in chapter 1. Add five incidents to it, however major or minor, that influenced your sexuality in ways that are related

to the issues in this chapter. Pick one of those new incidents, and write about it for ten minutes.

2. If you're impacted by social stereotypes about a particular part of your identity, spend at least thirty minutes researching people or organizations that are fighting back against that stereotype. What approaches appeal to you? What seems to be working? If you feel so moved, inquire into ways you can get involved in their work.

3. Take or draw a picture of a part of your body that you think looks great. Maybe you like the way your ankle curves from your calf into your foot. Maybe it's the feel of your skin, or the color of your eyes, or the strength of your shoulder. Whatever it is, show that part of you some extra love and attention. Stretch it, or rub in some oil, or spend ten minutes just admiring it. Then put that picture of it up somewhere where you'll see it at least once a day.

4. Write a poem about yourself.

5. Find delightful or annoying images of women, on the Internet or in newspapers and magazines. Stick them in your journal and give them a voice. Draw speech balloons and fill in the words they'd like to say. Let them talk back! Choose one of your women and write a story in which she over-turns the stereotypes people have of her.

6. Start with this line and continue writing: "I'm learning to . . . "

CHAPTER 4

A WOMAN'S INTUITION

YOU MAY BE SURPRISED TO HEAR THAT I'M A STAUNCH
defender of a girl's right to go wild. I just want to redefine
the terms under which we can do it. I think if you want to wear
a skimpy outfit because it makes you feel powerful or turned on,
then you deserve a world in which you can do that without being
harassed, shamed, or violated. If you want to make out with a
stranger on a dance floor because it's thrilling and feels a little
dangerous and because, well, that stranger is hot? Please get your
mack on. Ditto for flirting, being out alone after dark, drinking
socially, and nearly everything else on the list of things girls are
supposed to avoid doing lest we "get ourselves" raped. Because
you can't *get* yourself raped. No, really. You can't. Get yourself.
Raped. You can only *be* raped. And if someone is raping you?
Committing a violent felony assault against you? It's their fault,
not yours, regardless of what you were doing beforehand.

Now, let me take a moment to say that if you're not a wild
child by nature, by all means, stick to your nature. There's nothing liberating about acting like a party girl in order to prove

how free you are, when you'd rather be home in your jammies reading a book. What's more, few of us want the same level of wildness at all times. As long as you're doing what you enjoy, on your terms, and you're not hurting yourself or others in the bargain, there's no shame in wherever you fall on the snuggle-to-party spectrum.

So instead of adhering to a one-size-fits-none policy that discourages you from pursuing things you enjoy—whether it's skinny-dipping with friends or having a hot fling—why not develop the tools to listen to your own needs and boundaries, separate real danger from manufactured fear, and learn how to determine and weigh risks involved in any given situation?

But first, let's do a quick check-in: How's it going with the daily writing and the weekly body love? Are you doing it every day, never, or some of the time? How is it feeling? You're a quarter of the way through this book, and it's about to get a little more personal, so now is a great time to recommit to these tools, which are key ways to support and affirm yourself as you go through this process.

Dive In: To get in the mood, why don't you reread the list of body-loving activities you brainstormed in chapter 1, and then add a few more things to the list?

YOU'RE NUMBER ONE

The first and most important step in keeping yourself safe while pursuing a life full of pleasure is deciding that you are worth protecting. For many women, this is no small challenge. Critical to it is determining what your personal boundaries are and respecting them.

Boundaries—some people call them limits—are any point past which you're personally unwilling to go, or any behavior you're unwilling to put up with. You're the only person who can decide what your boundaries are, whether it's that you don't have sex until after the fourth date or that you feel like a particular person is being rude to you and you don't want to talk with them anymore. Your boundaries can change depending on who you're with and what mood you're in, and that's fine. What's important is that you learn what they are, and that they—and you—are worth sticking up for.

I tend to feel very selfish when I think about myself in any positive, want-to-take-care-of-myself kind of way. I have this feeling like "I don't deserve this. I don't do enough to deserve this." I tend to disassociate from my body, so I don't really know how to take care of my body, or know how to be good to my body, so I also tend to be like, Oh, well, if he doesn't want to use a condom, I'm sure it will be fine, even though I know that's really stupid. It just happens, and I regret it, and I beat myself up for it, but I think it does come down to thinking I'm not worth protecting or standing up for. I'm not worth questioning somebody else's decision. Like, what if this makes them not want me? {Heidi}

I've never felt clearer than when I admitted to myself out loud that if I don't care about myself, as a Black woman, nobody will. If I went missing, you wouldn't hear about me on the news. So when people are messing with me, I've decided to take the stance that I can be right, and our culture can be wrong. It is wrong. I'm not out of my mind, and it is within our power to change it. {Gray}

Taking care of your own safety should be one of your primary responsibilities. When I feel deserving of my personal boundaries and capable of defending them, I feel safer and more secure in my life, which frees up so much energy to focus on other things. I use a lot of that energy to work for the safety of other women. You can do amazing things with that energy, too, for yourself and other people you care about.

Dive In: Think about situations in which you've treated your needs or boundaries as unimportant. List at least five instances. Now pick one, and imagine that instead of you being in that situation, it had been someone you care about. Write an imaginary letter to that person, expressing what you wish they could have done differently in that situation. Acknowledge with compassion why it may have been hard for them to speak up for their boundaries, and then explain why it's so important to you that they overcome those obstacles and learn to believe and act like they're worth defending.

GETTING REAL ABOUT RISK

The first thing to know about risk is that it can't be avoided. There is no way to live your life completely and utterly safe from risk. Choosing to do nothing, ever, brings its own set of risks, including depression, vitamin D deficiency, muscle atrophy—you get the picture. And in terms of sexual safety, staying in your home certainly doesn't guarantee that no one will ever sexually violate you, given that most rapists choose victims they already know. So it's crucial to let go of the idea that there are choices you can make that will guarantee your safety. They just don't exist.

What *do* exist are different types of risk (the emotional risk of isolation vs. the physical risk of assault), different levels of risk (are you risking being rejected by someone you just met or having your heart broken by someone you love?), and related pleasures or other rewards associated with pursuing them (bonding with friends, sexual satisfaction, emotional intimacy, adrenaline rushes, etc.).

When it comes to assessing the risks associated with self-expression and sexuality, it's good to prepare in advance by separating myth from fact. Let's start by reality-checking some of the most common "risks" women are warned about:

Being Out Alone After Dark

Myth: A stranger will jump out of the bushes and attack you!
Reality Check: Could it happen? Sure. But it's pretty rare—around 80 percent of rape victims know their attackers, so, statistically speaking, you're in greater danger from the male acquaintance who offers to walk you home. Besides, men are 150 times more likely to be attacked in public by a stranger than

women are, so why is it that women are the ones taught to be afraid of being alone in public? Of course you should take precautions if you're in a particularly dangerous area, but overall, this myth doesn't make you safer—it detracts from the reality of how most attacks against women happen and makes women feel less free to live our lives.

> **Dive In:** Call your local police department and ask them how many violent crimes have been committed in your area, what percentage of the victims have been women, and how many of those were victimized while walking alone by themselves. (Keep in mind that 60 percent of rapes are never reported to authorities, and most of the nonreported ones are committed by someone the victim knows.) Then find out how many people have been injured or killed in car accidents in the same area in the same time period.
>
> Still don't feel safe? Be sure to read the section on self-defense later in this chapter.

Going Out Drinking

Myth: *It will get you assaulted! And it will make you slutty!*

Reality Check: For lots of people, including women, social drinking is fun. Sometimes it helps us loosen up in social situations, sometimes we simply enjoy the taste of great beer or cocktails, and sometimes we just like feeling a little buzz among friends. There's nothing wrong with that, as long as you're not regularly getting so hammered you can't think straight (in which case you may have a problem with alcohol).

However, it's important to know that alcohol and drugs are also the preferred tool of rapists. According to self-admitted rapists, over 70 percent used alcohol or drugs to subdue their victims.[2] So if someone you're with is *pressuring* you to drink or take drugs when you don't want to, that's a warning sign that you're not in good company. Even if this person is not a rapist, the fact that they ignore your reluctance to drink or your desire to stop means they're someone who doesn't respect your boundaries. Pretty self-centered company at best, really dangerous company at worst. (It bears repeating that it's still not your fault if you succumb to their pressure and then they assault you. No amount of alcohol or drugs can ever make getting raped your fault. But forewarned is forearmed.)

It's also utter bunk to suggest that drinking will give you sexual desires that you don't normally have when you're sober. It may reduce any resistance you might have to act on your desires, but it won't create desires in you that don't already exist. Think about it: You're probably not a thief. Does drinking make you more likely to steal? Not if you don't already have that impulse.

On the other hand, if you are deliberately getting drunk in order to do things sexually that you wouldn't do sober, that's not healthy or safe. Using alcohol or drugs to numb your own desires or boundaries can also numb the part of you that insists on safer sex, and it definitely numbs your intuition about whether or not a person is safe to be sexual with. Beyond that, getting drunk to override your sober judgment is a way of violating your own boundaries. Every time you do it, you're telling yourself: My boundaries don't matter. You're setting a dangerous precedent, because the next time someone ignores your boundaries, it will seem like less of a big deal, since you've done the same thing yourself.

> **≋ Dive In:** Not sure if you're crossing the line from healthy social drinking to a more dangerous cocktail? Ask yourself these questions:
>
> - Of the last (up to) five sexual encounters I've had, how many involved me being drunk?
> - Of the last (up to) five times I've had drunk sex, how many involved me doing something I regretted afterward?
> - When I think about having sex while sober, I feel _____.
>
> (I don't need to score this quiz for you, do I?)

Wearing Sexy Clothes/Being Flirtatious

Myth: People will assume you're "easy" or you "want it."

Reality Check: If people make assumptions about you based on how you dress, whether or not you like to flirt, or if you get down on the dance floor and make out with someone in public, that's their business. Just because you are expressing yourself sexually in public doesn't mean anybody has the right to expect that you'll take it further sexually with them or with anyone else who happens to be around. As stockbrokers say, "Past performance is not an indicator of future results."

Beyond that, research shows that predators look for targets that seem vulnerable. When you hear people say, "Rape isn't about sex; it's about power," that's what they mean. You can't "cause" someone to sexually abuse you by being too sexy. Sure, you may turn someone on enough that they'll try to hit on you for sex, but if they're not a rapist, they're not going to simply lose control and assault you. Sexy vs. modest isn't the distinction predators make. They're much more concerned with whether you look strong vs. whether you look vulnerable, and you can project either of these regardless of what you're wearing or who you're flirting with.

Might some people (who aren't dangerous) make assumptions about you if you're wearing something they consider "provocative"? Yes, that's a risk. As we discussed above, you weigh the risks with the rewards, and everyone's threshold is different. And perhaps your goal is to have others find you provocative. And that's okay, too. That doesn't give anyone the right to mistreat you, and it doesn't make you "easy." It simply makes you *you*.

On the other hand, if you're dressing or acting "sexy" because you think people will like you more, or for any reasons that have more to do with someone else's expectations than with what feels right to you, that won't get you any closer to what you really really want. In fact, the further you stray from your authentic self, the less likely you'll be to attract the kinds of people into your life that you genuinely want to meet.

I would rather be inside with apple cider and a copy of War and Peace. *That's just the kind of person I am. When I look at pictures of myself from several years ago, when*

*I was wearing the hair, and miniskirts, and stiletto heels,
you know, it was like my uniform—that was the fake part.
That was the inauthentic, here-I-am-performing-what-I-
think-sexuality-is part. It just wasn't natural to me. Which
isn't to say I'm not a sexual person. It just feels fake for
me to do that.* {Gray}

Also complicating the matter is the question of what, exactly, constitutes "sexy" behavior or dressing. Jessica Valenti, founder of Feministing.com, wound up in the center of a controversy when she wore a perfectly work-appropriate fitted sweater to a meeting with former president Bill Clinton, somehow inspiring a firestorm over how she used her breasts to draw attention to herself in the (incredibly tame) group photo taken at the event.[3]

On the other hand, some of us find that clothes that make us feel sexy fail to get read as such, even in settings where we really want them to: "Feeling sexy when you're buttoned up to the middle of your neck is really hard," says Enoch. "When I go to parties, I want to show more skin, but I also want to say, *Hey, look, I'm also trans.* We are told that the only way to feel sexy, as people with female-assigned bodies, is to show as much of that body as possible. It takes a lot of work to get out of that."

So have some fun. Play with your look and your behavior in ways that make you feel good, but try to let go of worrying "what people will think." Because you don't have any control over that anyhow.

Dive In: Declare Opposite Day. The idea here is to try something new in order to discover how well your current approach is working for you, or if another one might feel more true to yourself. There's no right answer—just notice whatever you learn.

If you usually dress in clothes that make you feel sexy (whatever those clothes look like to you—what matters is how they make you feel) when you go out socially, put on an outfit that mutes your sexuality the next time you go out. But if you usually are more low-key, put on an outfit that makes you feel sexy and go somewhere in it, projecting confidence. Either way, pay attention to how you feel as people respond to you. Do you feel more or less like yourself than you usually do?

Or put on your "Opposite Day" outfit and go somewhere in it acting as though you feel confident, even if you don't. Sometimes you fake it until you make it. And sometimes you discover you're not faking it as much as you thought you were. Notice how you feel as people respond to you. Does the outfit become more comfortable as you wear it, or less so?

Or put on your "Opposite Day" outfit and wear it around your house in private. Then, with the outfit still on, sit down and imagine wearing it somewhere public with confidence. Write about what it would feel like, and how you imagine people would respond to you.

Ultimately, what's important is knowing how to separate the real risks from the hype. And to learn how to evaluate your risk tolerance, which is unique to you. There's no mathemati-

cal formula to determine your limits, but there are three simple
questions you can ask yourself that always apply:

- *How bad will it be if this situation doesn't turn out*
  well? For example, if you've always wanted to try
  out a sex toy with your partner, and the worst-case
  outcome is rejection or social awkwardness, you
  may be more willing to do it, but if your partner
  wants to have unprotected sex, that can put you at
  risk of STDs (and possibly pregnancy), so you may
  be less willing to do it.

- *How good will it be if it goes my way?* Often when
  evaluating risk, we get caught up in the worst-case
  scenario. But it's important to also weigh the potential benefits if the risk pays off. Take relationships,
  for example. If there wasn't something worthwhile at
  stake—like pleasure, love, adventure, or intimacy—
  we wouldn't be tempted to take the risk in the first
  place. If the potential payoff means more to you, you
  may find you're more willing to take larger risks.

- *How likely is it that something bad or good will happen*
  if I do this "risky" thing? Using the information out
  there, as well as your own experience and the experiences of others you trust, make an assessment of
  how likely the outcomes are that you both fear and
  desire. Are there ways to pursue the rewards you're
  after without exposing yourself to these risks? Be
  sure to factor in things you can do to reduce risk,
  like always practicing safer sex or letting someone
  know where you're going and when to expect you'll
  return.

Dive In: List five sexual things that seem both risky to do and appealing to you. They can be things you've done before or things you've never tried—anything from going out in a hot skimpy outfit to asking a partner to tie you up to hooking up with a stranger. Now circle the one that's most appealing to you, and also circle the one that seems the riskiest (these may be different items on your list, or the same one). For each circled activity, ask yourself the three questions on the preceding page and write out your answers. List all the bad things that could happen if you do this thing (risks can be physical, emotional, financial, etc., and affect both you and other people); then assess how likely it is for those bad things to happen and think of anything you can do to reduce those risks. Then list all the potential good outcomes and assess how likely it is for them to happen. You don't need to make a decision about whether or not it's worth doing—just notice your feelings as you complete the exercise.

LISTEN TO YOUR INTUITION

A lot of times, we have to evaluate risks on the fly. That's when we have to rely on intuition.

We all have intuition. It's that funny feeling you get in your gut about something or someone when you don't really know why you have that feeling and yet there it is. Like when you know who's calling before you look at your caller ID. Maybe that feeling is saying, *Run away.* Maybe it says, *Go for it.* Maybe it says, *Proceed with caution.* Those are all messages your intuition can send you.

As women, we're taught to ignore our intuition. We're told it's a sign of weakness. But nothing could be further from the truth.

> I used to be a very intuitive person. I used to wear my emotions on my sleeve at all times. I just had a sense about things. But I got made fun of for being a crybaby or being too "out there," and so I began just keeping stuff inside, and that was around the time when my sense of noticing danger got warped. {Mag}

You may be wondering how the Terrible Trio fits in here. Fear, especially, can feel like intuition—and sometimes it is. Other times, it's been ingrained in us and is holding us back while masquerading as intuition. The best way to tell the difference between a helpful intuitive fear and a fake one that's holding you back is to practice. The more you practice listening to your intuition, the sharper it will become. The exercise at the end of this section will help you do that.

It's also worth checking out Gavin de Becker's book *The Gift of Fear*, which is a great source of information and inspiration on how to sharpen your intuition. De Becker—an expert security consultant—believes that our experience of intuition happens when our brain knows something and wants us to act so fast that it doesn't have time to explain to us why we know what we know. Here's what he has to say about it:

What [we] want to dismiss as a coincidence or gut feeling is in fact a cognitive process, faster than we recognize and far different from the familiar step-by-step thinking we rely on so willingly . . . Nature's greatest accomplishment, the human brain, is never more efficient or invested than when its host is at risk. Then, intuition is catapulted to another level entirely . . . Intuition is the journey from A to Z without stopping at any other letter along the way. It is knowing without knowing why.

Unlike generalized fear, which has only the loosest relationship with reality, *useful* fear is always specific. It says, *This particular person is lying to me. Don't go into that particular place right now. Let's get out of here.* Generalized fear can actually be dangerous, because it can be like the background noise at a loud restaurant, which keeps you from being able to hear the conversation you actually want to focus on. When you're afraid all the time, it's hard to hear a specific fear instinct, because the other fear buzzing inside you drowns it out. It may cause you to avoid ever learning enough about the situations you fear to develop the keen intuition that will help you navigate them safely.

Think about it this way: You know that sometimes people get into car crashes. If that knowledge developed into a fear of ever getting into a car, that wouldn't be intuition—it would be an overgeneralized fear that was holding you back from living your life. It would also make it harder to develop the real automotive intuition you need to keep yourself safe. Instead, if you learned more about the circumstances that made car crashes more or less likely and started by taking short, safer rides, working your way up to longer rides on faster roads at night, you would have the chance to develop your intuition about when a specific car was about to behave in a strange or dangerous way. And when you felt that intuition—a funny feeling that a car was about to swerve into your lane, though you couldn't say why—you'd be much safer if you listened and responded to it.

That said, your intuition can also be wrong, if it's based on inaccurate information. That doesn't mean you shouldn't listen to it in the moment. But it's useful to think about what triggered your intuition, after the fact. Did that man seem scary to you because he was wearing a heavy jacket in hot weather, and therefore might have been concealing a weapon? Or was he acting perfectly normal, but he was a man of color, and you've absorbed the false stereotype that men of color are more likely to be dangerous than white men? Checking the assumptions that underpin your intuition (after the fact, when you have time to think clearly) is an important way to make it more accurate, and to refuse to play into dangerous myths at the same time.

Dive In: Keep an intuition journal. This week, pay special attention to what your gut is telling you in different situations. They don't even have to be safety related. Maybe you'll have a twinge of a feeling that someone at your workplace is hiding something. Maybe you'll "just know" that your roommate or partner is lying to you when they say they already called the landlord as promised. Maybe you'll look at a car and know in advance that it's going to run a red light. Whatever your intuition tells you, make a note of it, and then note what you did in response to your intuition. Did you follow your gut, resist it, hesitate? When it's possible to know, note whether or not your intuition proved correct.

As you go, pick one or two intuitions and go a little deeper: In retrospect, why do you think you had that intuition? Can you identify the clues that you obviously knew but couldn't articulate to yourself at the time? Were they based on real information?

HOW TO SAY NO

Every time you listen to what feels like your intuition, you get better at separating the real instincts from the impostors. You build that muscle. And ignoring your intuition does the opposite thing. It's like a self-inflicted emotional injury. Make a habit of it, and it will leave your psychic immune system hobbled. And that leaves you vulnerable to manipulation, coercion, the Terrible Trio, and worse. Because when you regularly violate your own boundaries, it starts to seem like not such a big deal when someone else violates your boundaries. That's a downward spiral that leads to nothing good.

So let's get specific about how to take our intuition seriously. I know it can seem daunting to speak up for what you want and don't want, because many of us aren't in the practice of saying these sorts of things out loud. We've been taught that nice girls just don't. But expressing our needs doesn't have to be scary or hard—in fact, with some practice, it can be downright rewarding.

Let's start by talking about boundary setting, because one of the best ways to free yourself to say yes to what you want is to feel secure in your ability to say no to what you don't.

Say you're at a party. You're on the dance floor, getting your groove on, when a guy dances up to you. He's a friend of a friend—you were introduced to him briefly earlier that night. He starts trying to grind with you. It's nothing other couples aren't doing around you, but still you feel uncomfortable. Quick—what would you do?

_____

_____

_____

If you're like most women, you answered with some variation on "nothing." It's no mystery why: As women, we're taught from a young age to put other people's comfort ahead of our own. So in situations like this, we wind up thinking, *So he's dancing too close. It's not like he's hurting me or even saying anything weird. Besides, my friend knows him, so how bad can he be? It's not worth making a scene over.*

There are three dangerous assumptions in this line of reasoning:

1. *Any friend of my friend is a friend of mine.* Wouldn't it be great if this were true? Unfortunately, there are just too many variables here. How well do you know your friend? How well does your friend know this person? How much do you trust your friend's judgment about people? Always use your own judgment, not someone else's.

2. *My feelings are irrational and/or unimportant.* Along with learning to always put other people's comfort before our own, we're also taught that we're "irrational" and "overly emotional" and we need to keep our feelings in check. But if your gut is telling you something's not cool, and you try to silence that feeling because you're afraid people will think you're overreacting, you're shutting down the best first-response security system you've got. As de Becker writes in *The Gift of Fear,* "To override that most natural and central instinct, a person must come to believe that he or she is not worth protecting."

3. *Setting a boundary = making a scene.* It sure seems like this one is true, but if you're straightforward and respectful, it doesn't have to be. What's more, if someone causes a scene in response to your expressing a personal boundary, that's their fault, not yours, and it tells you something very important about their character.

Which brings us to the very simple yet powerful Nice Person Test. Here's how it works:

Imagine the roles are reversed. You're dancing with someone you just met at a party. Unbeknownst to you, you're getting too close and making that person kind of uncomfortable. Would you want them to tell you?

Of course you would, because you're a nice person. You don't want to make anyone uncomfortable—in fact, you probably would make some effort to put most people at ease. And you know what? Most other people are like that, too. So expressing your boundary in this situation is actually paying someone a compliment—it's treating that person as though you assume they are a nice, caring individual who wants you to be at ease. And if they behave otherwise, well, that tells you something crucial about that person, doesn't it?

Of course, how you express your boundary here is going to make some difference in how it's received, too. Here are two wrong ways to do it, and a right one:

- **WRONG: *Signs and Wonders.*** You don't want to come off as too aggressive, so you just take a step back to put some space between you, maybe excuse yourself to go to the bathroom and hope he'll be gone when you get back. It's a dangerous game—if this guy is bad news, he may be looking for signs that you're the "good" kind of victim who won't speak up for herself. You probably don't like to fail at much in life, but please, fail to be a good victim.

- **WRONG: *Preemptive Strike.*** You're so sure he's going to think you're a humorless bitch for wanting some personal space that you don't give him a chance to think otherwise, shouting at him something like, "You need to fucking step back, asshole." He certainly won't mistake you for an easy mark, but even if he is a nice guy, he may feel defensive and want to save face in front of his friends if he's suddenly getting reamed out by some girl about something he may not have even known he was doing. And then you will be causing a scene, which isn't fun for anyone and is going to make you more reluctant to express your boundaries in the future.

- *RIGHT: Nice and Direct.* The basic assumption of the Nice Person Test applies to how you express yourself, too. If you were in his shoes, what would you want to hear? How about a friendly but firm request like "Hey, we can keep dancing, but you're closer than I'm comfortable with. Can we make a little space?" Then smile warmly, continue dancing, and pay attention to what happens next.

Does he apologize and comply? Congratulations! You may well be dealing with a Nice Person.

Does he curse you out and walk away? Good riddance. Does he refuse to move, ignoring your request, mocking you for it or flatly declining it? Even getting more aggressively intimate than he was before? This is unlikely to happen, but if it does, it's an explicit threat. He is most definitely Not a Nice Person. Walk away from him (but don't turn your back on him entirely), flag down a friend or even a sympathetic-looking stranger, and together go safely to a different location that doesn't have him in it. If he follows you, or otherwise tries to prevent you from leaving, by all means, please make a scene. Directly and loudly tell individual bystanders what's going on ("This guy is following me and won't leave me alone!"), and if that doesn't shame him into backing off, ask someone to call 911. Would you rather be The Girl Who Overreacted at That Party That Time or risk being assaulted? I thought so.

Whatever happens, you'll have accomplished two important things:

1. You'll have learned crucial information about whether or not your new friend is a decent human being who respects your boundaries, and

2. You'll have prioritized your own intuition over your fear of offending or making a stir. That's an important part of overcoming some of the most toxic Girl Programming our culture dishes out. Prioritizing yourself is like working a muscle: Every time you do it, you'll make the next time easier and you'll feel more strongly that it's the right thing to do.

Dive In: Get out your notebook and spend ten minutes writing about a time you felt uncomfortable with someone's behavior toward you but didn't do anything about it. What were they doing and how did it make you feel? Why didn't you do or say anything? How did you feel about that person afterward? How did you feel about yourself afterward?

Now, spend ten minutes writing about the same situation, and imagine you applied the Nice Person Test and acted on it. What would you have done or said differently? How do you think the person might have reacted? How do you think you'd have felt about them afterward? How would you have felt about yourself afterward?

SELF-DEFENSE

Even the topic of self-defense can make people anxious. I know this because I taught it for years. So before we get into it, take a deep breath. Go ahead: in . . . out . . . Do it a few times if you need to.

The main reason women in particular feel anxious about self-defense is that it forces us to confront our vulnerability. I've heard from so many women and girls over the years who've said they were uncertain about taking the class because they were worried it would make them more afraid. They knew that they'd have to think about the scary possibility of someone committing violence against them, or that they'd have to remember violence they'd already suffered. They much preferred to just not think about it.

I have a lot of empathy for women who feel that way, and surely I never want to push someone into doing something they're not ready for. But I can tell you straight up that the role fear plays in my life is so much smaller now than before I learned to fight back. In other words, if you're trying to reduce the amount of energy you give to fear, the only way out is *through it.*

What do I mean by this? I'll tell you my story, and then we'll talk big picture.

I was sexually assaulted during my junior year of college. It was such an average portrait of how sexual assault happens, it's hardly worth describing—it was someone I knew; alcohol was involved; everyone wanted to know why I was making such a big deal out of it. But for me, it *was* a big deal. It was a rip in the fabric of my life—I suddenly understood that I wasn't safe in my own body. My body could be controlled by someone else just because he felt like it. It was . . . indescribable, honestly. It plunged me into a period of fear. I didn't want to hear any songs sung by men. If I was getting into an elevator on campus and there was an athletic-looking guy already on the elevator (the guy who attacked me was an athlete), I got off. I was afraid in public all the time, and it was exhausting. Not only had my security in my body been taken, but the amount of energy my fear now occupied was the ultimate insult added to my injury.

So when a friend of mine took a self-defense class that was then called Model Mugging (it's now called IMPACT in most places) and showed me the video of her "graduation," in which she took on gigantic padded assailants and fought them off with the power of a very focused tornado, I was transfixed. A month later, I was sitting in my sweatpants on a gym mat in a nondescript room, waiting for the first session to begin.

To say I knew nothing about self-defense would be an understatement. The sad reality was that the guy who attacked me was smaller than me. I now know that it would have taken very little to get him off me, to prevent all the trauma that I've suffered since. But I didn't know that then. All I'd ever heard growing up was the opposite message: *If a guy is trying to rape you, there's really nothing you can do. Don't fight back, or you'll just make him angrier.*

Now, this advice is completely, utterly bunk. Actually, it's worse than bunk—it's actively harmful. It's the opposite of what's true, and it puts women who follow it in much graver danger than they'd be in otherwise. In fact, researchers have discovered that women who fought back against would-be rapists not only were less likely to be raped, but, even if they were raped, had no more physical injuries than women who didn't try to defend themselves.[4]

But I knew none of that at the time. Not until the third class of IMPACT, the class in which we tackled what they call "reversals." They call sexual assault scenarios "reversals" because the strategy they recommend is all about reversing the script the assailant has in his head, and reversing the power dynamic of the situation.

Until that class, I'd been *loving* self-defense. Before IMPACT, everyone in my life had always told me to shush. I'm a loud girl by nature, so that's hardly a surprise, but damn if it didn't feel transformative for the IMPACT instructor to tell me to use my powerful volume on my own behalf. I'd also never hit another human being. (Well, maybe my sister when I was little, but I was never really trying to hurt her.) I'd certainly never hit another human being with my full force. I had no idea how hard I could hit! It felt amazing. I had never felt more powerful.

That all changed the moment I lay down on the mat and let the male instructor in his suit of padding, playing a potential rapist, climb on top of me. In that moment, the fire IMPACT had lit in my belly went out. I just couldn't put my heart into fighting him off. I went through the motions, yes, I even fought hard enough to "win," but it wasn't a win I could feel inside.

It took me a long while to figure out what the problem was. After all, I was ferocious when fighting in stranger-on-the-street scenarios, and I had so much more motivation to fight hard when it came to rape. What I eventually realized was this: I was afraid that if I knew now how to have prevented what happened to me then, I would no longer have the right to all of my feelings about what he did to me. It wasn't rational, of course, but trauma rarely is. It took me years to really find the fight in those reversals.

The other objection some women have to self-defense is that it puts the responsibility on women to protect themselves, instead of obligating rapists to not rape women in the first place. I'm pretty sensitive to this argument, having edited an entire book about how to stop making women responsible for rape prevention and to put the focus where it belongs: on the rapist. But advocating self-defense for women isn't about blaming current or future victims. It's about dealing with reality as it exists today.

The truth is, violence against women isn't going to end tomorrow. Realistically speaking, it's going to take decades (if not centuries) to undo all of the ways our culture encourages and allows rape. In the meantime, all the women living in the world are still, well, living. In the world. The current world, in which rape is shockingly common. Teaching women some tools we can use in case of emergency will help us deal with the world as it is while we're working to make it better.

Imagine we each have a toolbox in which we can store tools for keeping ourselves safe. In it, we've got condoms and dental dams, maybe, and good communication skills, self-awareness, safecalls (more on those calls in chapter 8)—you get the picture. Well, why *not* have some more tools in there as well? Doesn't having more tools make it more likely you'll have the one you need in an emergency?

Does that mean I'm never afraid for my safety? Of course not. But it happens a lot less often since I trained in self-defense, for a few simple reasons:

- I have much more information about how to assess any given situation and make an informed decision about how safe it is.

- If I feel afraid, I think about the worst thing that I'm afraid might happen, and then I calmly think through what my response would be. Knowing I can handle a worst-case scenario helps me let go of the fear and get on with my life.

Of course, self-defense isn't a silver bullet, and it won't make you invincible. There will always be the possibility that something will happen that you can't have been prepared to handle. But that likelihood will be much, much smaller if you get training. By the same token, however much training you have, you're under no greater obligation to fight back against an attacker than if you had no training. The act of rape is still their fault, never yours.

Dive In: During the next week, pay close attention to whether or not people's behavior is making you uncomfortable. Did your roommate borrow your sweater without asking? Did a coworker say something inappropriate? Is someone bumping into you unnecessarily on the train? Whatever the situation, ask them to stop their behavior using the Nice Person Test: Think about what you'd want to hear if you were in their shoes, and then say that. Notice your feelings before, during, and after you take action. Did you feel fear? Did you feel embarrassed? Did you feel relief? Did you feel excited or powerful? There's no right answer—it's just useful to notice how you feel when you start sticking up for your boundaries, so you can watch those feelings change over time as you get more and more practice.

Go Deeper: For some of you, this chapter may have stirred up uncomfortable memories. Most of us have experienced sexual behaviors that were unwanted, unpleasant, threatening, or downright abusive. You're probably thinking about some of those memories right now.

If it feels okay for you to write about one of these situations, you might find the advice below a helpful way to start. Choose any of them you like, and feel free to ignore the rest!

1. In your timeline, write a few incidents this chapter has reminded you of. Simply acknowledging your history can be a powerful act. You can always write more about any or all of them later if you want to.

2. Tell a friend or someone close to you that you are doing this work, so you don't feel you are alone. You can ask the friend to check how you're doing, or not. You can show them what you've written, or not.

3. Write in a café or somewhere else that has people in it. This can give you some human contact without its being intrusive.

4. Don't judge or edit your work. Just get it down, any which way. Keep the pen or keys moving. Don't go back and edit yourself.

5. Write in the mornings so that you don't go to bed with those bad memories.

6. Sneak up on it! Write around the edges. Write the landscape or the characters. Write other stories set around the same time. As you work in the "general area," you will become anesthetized to some extent.

7. Sometimes it helps to set a distance between you and the memories. Fictionalize. Change the point of view by writing about yourself as "she" or "you," rather than "I." Make it into a fairytale or a myth. Tell it from another angle—a tree, or an animal.

8. Write like a video recorder. Another way to get distance is to be coldly objective. Just write what happened, and don't even bother to say how you felt.

9. You can write and never share. You can keep the work absolutely private. You don't even have to read it yourself. Keep a secret journal or computer file only for that writing.

10. You can rewrite history. Write dialogues that address the conflicts, that tell people how angry or sad they made you feel. Take sections of

painful events and reshape them. Write better endings.

11. Remember positive influences. Focus on things that helped you survive, people who made a difference.

12. Build in a reward for when you're done—from ice cream to a walk with the dog.

CHAPTER 5

WHAT'S LOVE
GOT TO DO WITH IT?

I T'S IMPOSSIBLE TO WRITE A BOOK ABOUT SEXUALITY without talking about love, and I wouldn't want to even if I could. For many people, including me, sex as an expression of love is one of the most intimate and emotionally moving experiences we can have. It's far from the only healthy way to experience sexual interaction, but it can be a really great one.

There are all kinds of ways to think about sex and love. For some people, attraction and love are completely intertwined. These people can't conceive of being sexual with someone they don't love. For others, love and sex have almost nothing to do with each other. But these are the extremes—I suspect that most people fall somewhere in between. They experience love and sex as related but not exclusive to each other. Loving someone in a particular, intense way can make us want to be sexual with them, even if we wouldn't have otherwise been attracted to them. Some of us don't need to be in love with a person to have sex with them, but must at least have some basic respect or fondness for them. It can be any number of dynamics. The important thing is to figure out how *you* feel about the way love and sex interact in your life, not how others believe you should feel.

For Cassie, age thirty-eight, love came first, then attraction. "When I first met my husband, I had no interest in him whatsoever," she recalls.

I knew he was attracted to me and wanted to ask me out (he asked a friend of mine if he had a chance) and all I could think was, Oh, god. Really? Why him? I mean, I liked him well enough as a friend, but there was zero physical attraction to him.

Five years passed, and he was a groomsman in a wedding where I was a bridesmaid. We hadn't seen each other in the intervening five years, but that night we danced and talked and spent just about every minute with one another. Two years later we were married. And we're celebrating our sixth wedding anniversary this year.

I fell in love with him before I was attracted to him and, really, it's been the best thing ever. And now he's one of the sexiest guys I know.

The default assumption for girls and women is that we prioritize not just love but also relationships first, before sex, so we're willing to "give up" sex in exchange for commitment. That same model assumes that men want sex first and are sometimes willing to trade love and commitment to "get it." Of course, this model assumes that all women sleep only with men and vice versa, and that all people identify as either "men" or "women," so that should be a strong clue that this model is severely limited. At best.

The reality is that women—just like all people—vary quite a lot in terms of their sexual priorities. Further, unlike the model above, sex doesn't have to be a zero-sum game in which one person "gives it up" and another "gets it." Good, healthy sexual interactions give something positive to all participants. In other words: When sex is good, everyone's a winner.

But the kind of sexual contexts that leave us fulfilled are as varied as we are. Here are just a few examples of totally valid reasons to have sex with someone:

- Because you're in love and want to express and explore that love physically.

- Because you want to strengthen or celebrate an emotional bond you have with someone.

- Because you're horny and you're craving sexual release.

- Because you're sexually attracted to your partner.

- Because you love the afterglow.

- Because you're in a bad mood and it will cheer you up.

- Because you want to get pregnant.

- Because it just feels really good.

- Because it makes you feel calmer or more grounded.

- Because it's good exercise and relieves stress.

- Because it makes you happy to give your partner pleasure.

- Because partnered sex is spiritually important or satisfying to you.

These may not all be valid reasons for *you* to have sex. That's okay. The reality is, most of us don't have sex for all of these reasons, and often we prefer to have sex for a combination of these or other reasons. So maybe it's not enough that it feels really good, but in connection with an emotional bond, you can really get behind the pure physical pleasure as well.

 Dive In:

1. Make a list of reasons that seem like good ones for *you* to have sex.

2. Now, make a list of reasons that might seem good for other people to have sex, but not you.

3. Then make a list of what you think are generally bad reasons for *anyone* to have sex.

GOOD LOVE, BAD LOVE

Of course, in order to really figure out what you believe about the relationship between love and sex, you must first sort out what love means to you. (For the purposes of this chapter, we're talking about what's often called "romantic" love, to the exclusion of the kind of love you may have for your family, or your friends, or your pet, or for hot chocolate with fresh whipped cream.) Definitions of love vary widely across religions, cultures, and individuals, so once again, there's no "right" answer here. Just the one that makes sense for you.

Personally, I couldn't agree more with bell hooks when she writes, "The word 'love' is most often defined as a noun, yet all the most astute theorists of love acknowledge that we would all love better if we used it as a verb."

Sure, love has all kinds of ephemeral, emotional qualities, from the bordering-on-obsessive butterflies that come with new love to the deeply gratifying sense of peace that comes from forming a profound and stable long-term bond with a partner. For me, what really defines love is the consistent impulse to be loving to someone else in return. To actively support them, do my best to empathize with and understand them, and work toward their happiness, pleasure, and health. And that's also how I know if someone is loving me the way I deserve to be loved. Because we can't ever really know what someone is feeling. We can listen to what they're telling us—and believe me, I like to hear pretty words from my beloved—but in the end, if those words don't match up with consistently loving behavior toward me, it's not what I consider "real love."

Which gets to one of the trickiest parts of love—it's not always a two-way street. Love can be confusing and sometimes even scary. Because feelings aren't always voluntary, sometimes we fall in love with people who aren't safe or healthy for us to interact with sexually. And what do I mean by that? Well, these are people who consistently make us feel bad about ourselves. People who don't care about what we want—sexually or emotionally—or whether we're satisfied in bed. People who are careless with our safety, doing things like telling us they're monogamous in order to get us to forgo safe-sex barriers, while they're actually out sleeping with other people, potentially transmitting disease to us. People who will pressure us to do sexual things with them that we don't want to do at all, or don't want to do yet, or don't want to do with *them*. Even people who will ignore us when we set a clear boundary and force us to do things we've already said no to.

My friend Lila, thirty-five, learned this the hard way. "I was in a long-distance relationship and my boyfriend would expect that I would be available for phone calls whenever he was free, and I also had to be available completely whenever he was in town," she told me.

If I had plans, I had to go to untold lengths to twist myself in and out of an argument with him. He'd claim that I clearly had more important things to do than spend time with him; he claimed that I was the most important thing on his agenda, so why wasn't he my most important thing? Somewhere in my head, I knew it was a Bad Thing, but something about being in this deeply intimate yet distant relationship made me make all kinds of excuses. In retrospect, I'm still beating myself up for "letting" him treat me that way. I consider myself a pretty badass feminist, and I know that I shouldn't be ashamed, but I am.

Unfortunately, some people will also use love as a weapon against you. They may say some version of, "If you loved me, you would do it." When you try to leave them because they're treating you badly, they'll tell you how much they love you, and how no one will ever love you as much as they do. Or they'll tell you they need your love, that your love is the only thing keeping them going, or the best thing that's ever happened to them, and therefore you just *can't* leave them.

The thing is, it may be absolutely true that you feel love for someone and are driven to act lovingly toward them, and yet they can also be bad for you. Loving someone—and even having that person say they love you back—doesn't mean the relationship is healthy or good for you, or that you "owe" them anything, sexually or otherwise. Contrary to the myth you get sold by Hollywood and the music business, love doesn't conquer all, and it's not going to protect you if the person you love is treating you badly or hurting you. Don't ever let your love for someone else be more important than your love for yourself. You can love someone and still need to stay away from them, or leave them. It happens all the time. If you're at all confused about whether someone you love or who claims to love you is treating you badly, here are a list of signs to watch for (adapted from Heather Corinna's book, *S.E.X.*):[1]

- You're putting other important relationships or goals of yours at risk because of the relationship.

- You're becoming isolated from everyone but your partner.

- You're making a lot of excuses for your partner.

- You're feeling sad, frustrated, or upset with your relationship or your sexual encounters far more than you find yourself feeling happy.

- You're using sexual activity or other behavior to avoid or defuse relationship conflicts, or "zoning out" during sex.

- You're having trouble discussing, making, or enforcing limits and boundaries (sexual or otherwise) with your partner.

Ultimately, if sex feels too intimate or sacred to share with a relative stranger, that's a great reason to reserve sex for people you love. Believing that love will keep you safe from violence or heartbreak is not. The reality is, love is no guarantee against either possibility.

Getting clear about your own beliefs about love may help you get clear about which love is good for you and which love isn't. It can also help you understand what's best for you when it comes to love and sex.

> **Dive In:** Create your own definition of love. How can you tell (or how do you think you would be able to tell) if you are in love with someone? How can you tell if someone loves you? What does healthy love feel like, and how does it make you (and people who feel it for you) act? What does love always involve? What does love never involve?
>
> Once you've written your definition, write a list of the people you've been in love with, or who've said they were in love with you. Think about those relationships. How well do they match your current definition of love?

WHAT ABOUT LOVE HORMONES?

You may have heard about oxytocin. It's a chemical that is often released during sexual stimulation. Some studies have shown that when we release oxytocin, it can intensify the feelings (both positive and negative) we have about the person we're having sex with. Unfortunately, this chemical response has been warped into an argument by abstinence-until-marriage advocates and other social conservatives, who claim that because of this bond, women get hurt by casual sex more than men.[2] And the argument goes further, claiming that if women form an oxytocin bond with too many people, the effect will wear off and they'll find themselves unable to bond properly with anyone.[3]

Please.

The truth is, there is still a lot to understand about the role oxytocin plays in our lives. Like any hormone, it's one ingredient in the stew we call our emotional behaviors—it's pretty hard to separate it out once it's mixed in. But I'll leave it to the professionals, like the American Psychological Association, to clarify this. They spotlight a study of prairie voles, in which researchers compared the stress reactions of female prairie voles living for four weeks either in isolation or with a female sibling and found greater levels of stress, behavioral anxiety, and depression in those separated from their siblings. The team then gave the animals either oxytocin or saline every day during the last two weeks of the four-week period. The isolated animals treated with oxytocin no longer showed signs of depression, anxiety, or cardiac stress. By contrast, oxytocin had no measurable effects on those paired with siblings, suggesting that "the effects of oxytocin are most apparent under stressful conditions."[4]

In other words? Too *little* oxytocin early on can be damaging, but too much? No such effect has been found.

What's more, oxytocin is produced in a wide array of situations, many of which have nothing to do with sex. Heather Corinna, writing at Scarleteen.com, summarizes these conditions below. And her facts check out.

- for people with a uterus, during labor (a synthetic version of oxytocin, Pitocin, is often used to induce labor), birth (vaginal delivery), and/or breastfeeding

- when men snuggle babies

- when we pet or look at our dogs

- during massage (from anyone, but found to elevate more in the massage therapist than the massagee)

- when we sing together in groups

- when we compete, play games, or gamble

- kissing (though this apparently raises men's levels more than women's)

- hugging

- acupuncture

- talking intimately with your friends, apparently especially between female friends

- yoga, meditation, or prayer

- some foods, like chili peppers, which contain a compound called capsaicin, which has been shown to prompt a surge of oxytocin

If our ability to bond with others wore down every time we engaged in one of these activities, the whole human race would be pretty antisocial by now, wouldn't we?

So don't worry: Even if you have multiple sex partners, you'll never become like an unsticky piece of tape. Bond away, however and with whomever you like.

> **Dive In:** Not convinced? Want to learn more so you can explain the issue to others? Do yourself a favor and go read Heather Corinna's entire Scarleteen.com article separating oxytocin myth from fact: www.wyrrw.com/scarleteenoxy.

MONOGAMY VS. POLYAMORY

One of the major questions to ask yourself about how you want love and sex to interact is a question that I suspect most people never consider: Do I prefer monogamy or polyamory?

Let's start by defining some terms. Monogamy is generally understood to be a relationship model in which two people commit to being sexual and romantic with each other exclusively, often forever. Monogamy has a lot of powerful advocates: Many religions believe it's the only "right" way to have a romantic and sexual relationship, and Western governments, at least, give it a whole lot of help by creating marriage policies that make it easy for monogamous (heterosexual) couples to gain access to all kinds of benefits that are otherwise hard or impossible to get.

Monogamy works for a lot of people. When practiced thoughtfully, it can create feelings of stability and trust and, in comparison with polyamory (more on that in a bit), can help partners minimize feelings of jealousy. Of course, any romantic and sexual relationship—whether monogamous or not—takes a lot of work at least some of the time, and monogamy means that you have only one relationship to nurture. Unfortunately, it's often practiced thoughtlessly (and therefore poorly). And it's not the only relationship option that can work.

Polyamory generally describes a romantic relationship in which partners are free to form sexual and/or emotional relationships with other people as well. Depending on how it's practiced, those relationships may all be considered equal, or there may be a "primary" relationship that takes precedence over "secondary" relationships. These secondary relationships may be primarily sexual, or they may involve deep emotional bonds and commitments. There may also be a "primary" relationship among more than two people—that is, one form of polyamory involves three or more people, all primarily committed to each other as partners.

Polyamory—not to be confused with polygamy, an often misogynist arrangement in which a man has several wives, usually subservient to him—is a new idea to a lot of people, but it's hardly a new practice. People have been doing it in one form or another for centuries. It can get complicated—polyamory provides more opportunities to grapple with jealousy; plus, with every new person comes new challenges, such as finding communication styles that work for you both, coordinating schedules, and learning how compatible you are with each person's needs, desires, and boundaries, and not everyone is up to those challenges. But it can also be very rewarding, encouraging self-discovery, empathy, and explicit communication and providing feelings of both community and personal autonomy that can be harder to come by with monogamy. And it rarely gets boring.

Enoch explains,

What I love about polyamory is that it takes a lot of the un-fun urgency out of relationships. We get to enjoy the places where our needs and desires overlap and don't have to panic if there are places where they don't. If one of us has needs that the other can't fulfill, we can get them served elsewhere, and it's okay. We can relax and focus instead on the fun types of urgency that come with connecting with people on various levels.

Neither monogamy or polyamory is a good excuse to avoid the direct, ongoing communication necessary to sustain a healthy relationship, but both are too often used as such, in different ways: Monogamists often rely on assumptions about what "the rules" are (for example, what counts as "cheating"? Is flirting okay?) without ever discussing them, only to discover when someone gets hurt that both partners weren't operating with the same assumptions. And polyamorists sometimes throw themselves into the distraction of a new relationship instead of dealing with issues that need to be resolved in their existing one(s).

So, if neither approach is without risk (because what's without risk?), and both offer different benefits, it all comes down to what you really really want. Depending on your background, this may be a strange question, because many of us have never been offered an option besides monogamy. But it's a key one to consider, because it's much easier to manage the difficulties of whatever option you choose when you know you've chosen it freely and consciously.

> ≋ **Dive In:** Imagine yourself practicing the healthiest version of monogamy you can envision. What does your best vision of monogamy include? Do the same for polyamory. Now, using images, colored paper, fabric, or whatever materials you like, make two different collages expressing how those ideal visions of monogamy and polyamory might feel.

HOOKING UP

I'm going to say something now that may sound shocking, so brace yourself: There's nothing intrinsically wrong with "hooking up." Nothing. Nada. Not even if you're a girl.

Don't get me wrong: There's nothing intrinsically awesome about hooking up, either. It depends on what you're into. What do I mean by "hooking up"? It's when you have sex with someone for the fun of it, with no strings attached, no promise of or interest in nurturing a relationship. Just feel-good sex. For some people, attraction and affection are completely intertwined to the point where they can't be separated, and for others they have little to do with each other. The important thing is not to make assumptions or judgments about whether hooking up is acceptable, for yourself or anyone else.

In fact, in 2009, researchers at the University of Minnesota interviewed over 1,300 sexually active young adults between the ages of eighteen and twenty-four about their last sexual encounter, and then assessed their emotional well-being. Guess what? The 20 percent who had last gotten it on with a casual partner were no more emotionally damaged than the 80 percent who had most recently played with a committed partner. They weren't more depressed, and they had just as much self-esteem.

Buffy, age twenty-six, is a great example of this: "To date, my most satisfying and liberating experience was my first casual hookup," she told me.

It was after a tough breakup, and I was feeling hopeless. I didn't think I would ever be desirable again, and I wasn't sure if I would experience sexual pleasure again. I was wrong. Those orgasms I had left me high for days, and I felt more confident than any boyfriend had ever made me feel. It also prepared me to continue experiencing pleasure on my own terms, and now I don't settle for anything less.

So why the constant freaking out about "hookup culture"? Why the endless news reports and articles and books worrying about the fate of girls who engage in casual sex? And why do we never see the same hand-wringing about boys who sleep around?

There are a few overlapping reasons, but we have to start, of course, with the pervasive cultural double standard that says women want love and are willing to "give" sex to get it, while men want sex and are willing to "give" love to get it. This is pretty gross and insulting to everyone involved. Are we all so one-dimensional that we can want only one thing at a time? And are there really no men who prioritize love over sex, or women who do the reverse? And even if men are more likely to prioritize sex, and women are more likely to prioritize love, isn't it likely that this is a self-fulfilling prophesy? I mean, if the culture's telling you from day one that if you're a woman, love should be more important to you than sex, and furthermore employing the Terrible Trio to scare you off any sexual feelings you do have, is it any wonder if you wind up thinking love is more important to you than sex?

Of course, by this point you've begun to turn the volume down on those influences, but let's not forget that most people haven't. So if you act in ways that fly in the face of that "women = love"/"men = sex" standard, it can seem very dangerous and unnatural to people watching from the outside. It's true that some of the loudest public voices (from conservative politicians to religious-right media pundits and lobby groups) screaming that the sky is falling because of "hookup culture" are actively dedicated to controlling women through our sexuality. But it's also true that a lot of other folks (like everyday parents and teachers and community leaders) who share that worry mean very, very well. They just don't have the information you have.

But there's more to the hookup conversation than just slut-shaming, and some of those well-meaning social critics have decent points to make. They're worried about the role alcohol plays in hookups (we talked about alcohol and sex in chapter

4). They worry that girls who hook up with guys aren't doing so on their own terms, and believe they're being manipulated into sex by guys or they're having it because they believe it's the only way to get a guy's attention.

These are perfectly legit concerns. The only problem is, they have nothing to do with whether or not sex is casual or committed. Do guys never sexually manipulate women in the context of a relationship? Do girls (or guys, for that matter) never get hammered in order to suppress their own inhibitions when they're dating someone long-term? When we say, "I'm worried about girls hooking up" instead of, "I'm worried about people having drunk sex, and also about unequal gender dynamics in relationships," we accomplish two things, neither of them good. We fail to talk about the actual problems that we're worried about, and we add fuel to the slut-shaming fire that's already raging in our culture.

We also buy into the fallacy that women who hook up are ruining their chance at a "real" relationship.

Research just doesn't bear this out. A 2010 study by Anthony Paik at the University of Iowa found that the number one predictor of whether or not a new pairing resulted in a long-term relationship was whether or not both people in the pair were looking for a long-term relationship. Even those who had sex on the first date had an equal chance of going the relationship distance, as long as both people were looking for a marathon, not a sprint. So if you're looking for a marathon, be sure to go to bed with other marathoners. And if all you're looking for is a sprint, you're not going to be much worried about your marathon time, are you?

Dive In: Write a story about a woman who has casual sex and nothing bad happens to her as a result. It could be you or someone you know or someone made up—the story can be based on something that really happened or entirely invented. She can face unrelated challenges, if you like (it's hard to write a story with no conflict!), but in the course of the story, she should hook up with someone casually, have a great time, and face no bad consequences.

UNEQUAL DESIRES/EXPECTATIONS

Most people, when they talk about hookups, think that girls who participate in them are "settling"—that they obviously really want a relationship but aren't pressing for one because they think a hookup is all they can "get" from the boy they're with. (This whole social hand-wringing over hookups assumes heterosexual pairings, of course.) And that happens, for sure. We still live in a sexist, unequal culture in which boys and men have more social power than girls and women, and that means that often, women are expected to put our desires and needs aside in order to cater to the needs and desires of the men we want to be with. That's real. And it needs to stop.

But that's not the *only* way unequal desires rear their ugly heads. The truth is, this same sexist culture puts pressure on men to want *only* no-strings sex, which means that they may want something more but feel too worried that their masculinity will be questioned to say so. And certainly there are plenty of women who like casual sex, whether as a regular practice or as a once-in-a-while indulgence. Which is to say nothing of folks who don't fit the gender binary, or who are sleeping with same-sex partners, and may feel a huge cultural silencing bearing down on them as they struggle to tell their partner what they want.

Basically, the old saying is true: When you assume, you make an ass out of "u" and me. And if you're going to hook up, the only way to reduce your emotional risk is to get real about what you want from the experience. Monica, age twenty-two, told me about a situation she got into with a guy:

We were both into hooking up casually, but still had a huge miscommunication that ended in a lot of hurt feelings, especially on my part. I was very inexperienced and into the idea of hooking up fairly regularly, but he just didn't have the kind of time I was hoping for. I knew he had multiple partners, but he didn't tell me until long after I would have liked that he was really into someone on an emotional level and wanted to be spending a lot of time with her. I felt like I had been acting like a huge ass, pursuing him when he really wasn't into it, because I didn't have all the facts.

That question starts with you: Before you hook up with someone, do a gut check. How are you going to feel about this before, during, and after it happens? What if you never see this person again, or see them with someone else tomorrow? Would that really be cool with you? If it might feel bad, how bad would it feel? Is that a risk you're willing to take?

> ≋ **Dive In:** Think about a time when you've
> either been hurt or hurt someone else emotionally
> because of unmatched expectations from a sexual
> encounter. (If this has never happened to you, imagine
> a situation in which it might happen.) Now go back and
> think of a point leading up to that sexual interaction when
> you could have checked in about your expectations and
> possibly avoided some of those hurt feelings. Once you've
> identified your moment, literally rewrite the script: Write
> down what you could have said differently to clear the air
> in advance. Then write your partner's imagined response.
> Work out the whole dialogue. How does it turn out?

FRIENDS WITH BENEFITS

Here's the most popular argument against "friends with benefits" (FWB) arrangements: They don't last. Someone starts feeling romantically attached, and then it all goes to hell.

That's possible. It certainly happens in some FWB arrangements, though I don't know what percentage because I've never
seen a study of it. But let's assume we can even say this happens in most FWB arrangements. My reply would still be the
same: Some romantic relationships go to hell at one point or
another, too. I'm not trying to be harsh, but it's a fact. In the
United States, approximately 43 percent of first marriages end
in divorce,[5] and that's counting only the people who made it far
enough in the relationship to decide to give marriage a go. So
to single FWB relationships out as emotionally risky in some
special way is unreasonable. All relationships are emotionally
risky in one way or another.

The truth is, there are any number of good reasons to acquire a friend with whom you also share sexual "benefits." Maybe you're at a critical moment in your education or career and don't have the time and energy required to sustain a deep romantic involvement, but you don't want to be celibate, either. Maybe you met someone and have decided they're not a long-term match for you, but you're still really attracted to them and like them as a person. Maybe you're not ready for a deep relationship because you're still healing from one emotional wound or another. Maybe you want a committed relationship but haven't found the right person yet and want some companionship while you continue looking. It hardly matters why. What matters is that it works for you and that your FWB partner is on board with the arrangement as well, like in the case of Bobbie, age forty-nine:

My best friend and I did one another on the regular when we were in between relationships. I loved her and she loved me, we knew we weren't right for each other as far as a long-term relationship, but we loved fucking one another. She was a great lover and we were great friends. It worked for us for several years, until I moved away.

What's more, when they work, FWB relationships have several practical advantages over onetime hookups. Because you're having sex with the same person over and over, you're bound to become better lovers for each other. Plus, it's often easier to negotiate safe sex and prevent STDs when you're with the same person over time. And let's not forget the friendship part: Whether you started as friends and then introduced benefits or developed a real friendship through postplay pillow talk, the emotional intimacy of a real friend with benefits can be comforting and satisfying. I've cried in front of FWB partners, gotten great career advice from them, taken them to fancy-dress parties when I needed a date, snuggled all night with them when I needed comfort, and celebrated big moments together—none of which I'd do with a random hookup.

The only reasons to steer clear of FWB relationships are if you're not comfortable with them in general or if one of you actually wants something more.

Dive In: Complete the following sentences:

A good friend always _____

A good friend sometimes _____

A good friend never _____

A good lover always _____

A good lover sometimes _____

A good lover never _____

DEALING WITH HEARTBREAK

This isn't a book about love or relationships, but it's impossible to talk about the fullness of sexual intimacy without talking about emotional intimacy, too. And when we talk about emotional intimacy, we have to talk about heartbreak.

There's no way around it: Heartbreak sucks. If it didn't, we wouldn't have named it a word that suggests that the most crucial organ in your body is failing. The pain can be that intense. And there's nothing I can say to make that pain go away. But there are a few things I've learned that can help ease it a little:

Be Gentle with Yourself

Sure, that means lie on the couch and eat ice cream and watch your favorite show on DVD for days on end, or whatever your version of that is. But think about that when it comes to your sexuality, too: Don't expect too much too soon. Maybe you feel regret or pain about what you did or didn't do with your partner sexually. Maybe you just have to grieve the loss of a trusted partner you shared that part of yourself with. Give it time. As tempting as it may seem to "get right back on the horse" (ahem), make sure you're checking in with yourself to make sure it's what you really really want before you put yourself out there again sexually. Otherwise, you'll just wind up feeling worse than when you started. Which brings me to:

Feel Your Feelings

What terrible advice, right? I mean, who wants to feel these awful feelings? Isn't it better to shove them down into some dark internal corner and pretend you're Just Fine, Damnit? Well, your mileage may vary, but I say no. In my experience, the best way to get through painful feelings is to feel them. When you shove them aside, they fester and rot and infect other parts of your life, and eventually come back up again much worse than they would have been the first time around. Instead, allow yourself to feel however you feel. If you feel broken, feel broken. If you feel angry, feel angry. If you feel desperately sad, feel desperately sad. If you feel secretly relieved, feel secretly relieved. Don't judge your feelings or try to change them. Just feel them. And don't worry—they may feel like they'll be around forever, like this is the new permanent state of affairs for you emotionally, but it's not true. Every feeling passes and changes and evolves. The good ones do—no feeling of glee or joy or satisfaction lasts forever without interruption. And so do the bad ones. All feelings change over time. Let them do their thing. We'll talk about working with your feelings more in chapter 6, but if you need help surviving them, please also lean on friends and family, get mental health care if you can, and check out Kate Bornstein's book *Hello, Cruel World: 101 Alternatives to Suicide for Teens, Freaks and Other Outlaws*—a very accepting and creative resource for dealing with painful feelings of all kinds.

Learn, but Don't Overgeneralize

Every one of my heartbreaks has had something to teach me. Some of them have taught me about the dangers of allowing myself to see only the good parts of my beloved's behavior. Some of them have taught me not to compromise too much of myself in a relationship, and some of them have taught me that it's equally damaging to refuse to compromise at all. Some of them have taught me that two good people can love and even like each other and not be a good match for a long-term partnership.

It's natural to want to make meaning out of pain. To imagine we're suffering for no reason at all makes it feel worse. But there's a difference between looking for useful lessons from heartbreak and creating more of that generalized fear we discussed in chapter 4.

Consider the compromise issue. In some of my early adult relationships, I compromised myself almost absolutely, because I have a generalized fear of being abandoned and I thought if I always pleased my partners, they would never leave me. Turns out, that approach doesn't actually prevent anyone from leaving—and even if it did, it makes for a miserable relationship and a miserable life. But when I finally figured that out, I created from it a generalized fear of compromising with my partner. Guess what? Being an unyielding narcissist doesn't make for happy relationships or a happy life, either.

So take what you can from your experiences with heartbreak, yes. But be careful not to take too much, or you'll wind up letting it define you. Don't create new generalized fears that make it hard to hear your intuition—and hard to find the love you want and deserve.

Dive In: Write a letter to someone who broke your heart. Tell them what you learned from your relationship together, and from the way it ended. Get as specific and practical as you can about how you'll be (or already are) applying these lessons—"I learned to pay attention to whether or not someone's actions match up with their words" is better than "I learned not to trust liars." If it feels authentic, thank your heartbreaker for teaching you these lessons, and also let them know ways in which you've let go—that you're not letting the experience define you.

In all of these choices, keep in mind that your decisions don't have to be all or nothing. You can choose to be sexual in different ways with different people at different times in your life, or in different situations. You may want committed monogamy now because it feels right with your current partner, but then choose to pursue casual sex if you break up, then later enter into a polyamorous arrangement because that feels right to explore at the time. The point is, your desires about sex and relationships may be fluid, and it's okay to mix it up, as long as you're expressing your authentic desires.

You may also try out new styles of sexual connection and discover they don't feel right to you—and that's okay. As long as everyone is being safe and respectful, it's not the end of the world to take a risk and have it not work out. (More on this in chapter 7.) The point is to know what your options are and how to make the best decisions for yourself in the moment.

Go Deeper:

1. Add to your timeline examples of different sexual relationship models you've tried. Pick two different ones and write about what parts of them were fulfilling or fun, and what parts were difficult or painful.

2. Describe the perfect sexual relationship(s) for you right now. Get specific. What are your perfect partner or partners like? What rules or agreements make the arrangement feel so good? What, if anything, have you promised yourself or your partner(s)? How do you behave toward each

other when you're not having sex? And when you
are? What is the actual sex like? How do you feel
about each other? How do the relationship(s)
make you feel?

3. Make a map of your relationships. You are the
circle in the center, and your friends, lover(s), and
relatives are like the planets that circle around
you. The nearer you put them, the closer you feel
to them.

4. List the top thirty things that you need/want
from others, from emotional support to specific
sexual needs, from someone who brings flowers,
to someone who'll clean the toilet once in a while.
What do people do for you to make you feel
happy, healthy, and fulfilled (and yes, it's often a
two-way process)? Number the list.

Match numbers up with people. Who's doing
what when it comes to relationship needs?

Write in your journal about any surprises or
insights you may have had during this exercise.

CHAPTER 6

FREAKS AND GEEKS

W ELCOME TO THE SECOND HALF OF THE BOOK! HOW are you doing so far? Are you taking care of yourself, reaching out to positive supports in your life? Keeping tuned in to yourself through the daily writing, and exploring and affirming your right to pleasure through the weekly body love?

To whatever extent you are, great. And if you're struggling with any of it, that's okay, too. Don't use this process to beat yourself up, please. *Do* use it to challenge yourself, to explore uncomfortable or even painful places in the interest of getting to what you really really want. If your internal critics get too loud, go back and reread the commitment you made to yourself at the beginning of this process. Remind yourself of what's important here. But don't make yourself feel bad. Because there are plenty of people and forces in the world who are too happy to do that work. Don't help them.

Which brings me to the theme of this chapter. Whether in terms of the kind of sex we want to have, our sexual orientation, our "unconventional" body, a special ability or disability, a mental health issue, or anything else that violates people's expectations of how a woman should look or behave, many of us feel like freaks and geeks in one way or another. I assure you, if you do, too, you are far from alone.

Oppression and discrimination are real and are reinforced every day by the most powerful institutions in our culture: the mass media, organized religion, medicine, governmental agencies, the legal system, and more. If you've internalized the belief that there's something "wrong" with or "undesirable" about you, it's probably because the world you live in sends you that message on a daily basis. That can make the freaky feelings painful and hard to overcome, but it doesn't make them true. And there are things you can do to turn the volume down on them.

Starting in chapter 7, you'll be focusing your attention on how to interact with others, how to ask them for what you want and tell them what you don't want. How to build the partnered sex life you want. How to talk with friends and family about their role in supporting your healthy sexuality. And how to be a good partner, as well as friend and family member, to others. Probably, these are things you're eager to delve into.

But healthy sexuality has to start with you. If you don't believe in your own right to pleasure, your own desirability, and your own ability to give yourself pleasure, all of your interactions with others will be on their terms. Believe it or not, this chapter—the one about feeling too weird to be worthy—is your deep breath. A chance to get grounded and centered in your own sexuality before you invite anyone near it. And you may be guessing some of what that means: masturbation.

Stop for a second and check in with your body. How does that word make you feel? Excited, anxious, self-conscious, ashamed, aroused, repulsed? Masturbation can stir up some strong feelings, as Bobbie knows all too well:

I was raised as a strict Catholic in Boston. Around the age of nine or ten I began to fantasize about being kidnapped by women on horseback, and I rode out that fantasy through masturbation within the confines of my bathroom. We were always taught that what you did in the dark would show up in the light, so you can imagine my surprise after masturbating one day to find a stain in my panties. I promised God I would stop doing what was so obviously wrong if He would not tell my mother. The stain went away, but the desire didn't. I did my own laundry to hide my shame and kept up the masturbating, thinking I had gotten away with it. I woke up one morning after a particularly good masturbation the night before to find blood everywhere in my bed. God was going to make me confess! Until my menses ended some forty years later, I was always hottest when my period came around.

It's amazing how loaded the subject of masturbation can be, especially considering that it's probably the least controversial sex act imaginable: It carries zero risk of disease or pregnancy or coercion, and a low risk of injury unless you're doing something fancy. Since it doesn't involve another person, you don't have to worry about communication issues or whether or not your partner will respect you in the morning. And talk about enthusiastic consent! It's not like you're going to do it to please anyone besides yourself.

Maybe you've been masturbating since you were a child, and you've never *not* loved it. That's awesome.

But still, masturbation is like the third rail of sex talk, especially when it comes to the subject of Girls Who Do It. Is there any clearer evidence that we still live in a culture that's profoundly confused about female sexuality when it's easier to talk about porn than about self-pleasure? Amazingly, the idea that we women not only have our own real desires, but can also satisfy them ourselves, still can seem shocking and disturbing to mainstream society.

Which is precisely my point: Masturbation is a powerful experience and one of the most central ways to explore what you really really want. So let's bust some myths about it and send the Terrible Trio packing.

Myth: If you're in a monogamous relationship, masturbation is the same as cheating.

Reality Check: Look, I'm not going to tell you what rules to set up in your own relationship. But I wouldn't ever want to be in one where self-love was considered competition for partnered sex. First of all, in every relationship, libidos ebb and flow— your partner isn't going to be able to meet your every need at every moment. And if you've agreed not to seek sexual satisfaction with other people, why shouldn't you at least be able to scratch your itches yourself?

But honestly, my defense of jilling off, even when in a relationship, goes deeper than that. This is about you and your right to have whatever relationship with your body you want to—regardless of whether or not you're in a relationship that involves somebody else's body. Masturbation during a monogamous relationship is perfectly healthy and quite common, and it can go far in improving your sex life. Being practiced in what makes your body feel good, you'll know how to direct your partner during sex together. If you need help in figuring out how to have a frank and open discussion about sexuality with a partner, no worries—we'll get to that in chapter 7.

Myth: *Only boys masturbate.*

Reality Check: Historically, masturbation has been viewed as a coming-of-age milestone for boys, but not for girls. Quite the reverse, actually—in Victorian England, a woman who orgasmed was considered a sexual deviant. Thankfully, we've come a long way since then. A 2008 study out of the United Kingdom found that 92 percent of the eighteen- to thirty-year-old women surveyed masturbate, and over 65 percent do it two or three times a week. So when I say you're not alone? You really aren't.

Facts aside, there's nothing that will convince you quite like trying it. So let's talk about how to do it.

Let me start by telling you a little story to settle your nerves. I had a boyfriend in high school who loved me very much, and whom I loved back just as much. We lusted after each other constantly and fooled around whenever we could. And, as luck would have it, he was nearly as invested in my pleasure as he was in his own. (This is a great quality in a partner—don't leave home without it.)

Why am I telling you this? Because I never had an orgasm with him. I faked it constantly, because I knew it was important to him that I had them. But I didn't know how, and I was too embarrassed to say so. Besides, I was having a great time in bed with him, and I didn't know what I was missing, so I didn't miss it. So I lied. Over and over and over again.

We broke up when he went off to college, and then I went to college, too. I fooled around with a number of guys, but still— no orgasm. I'd given up trying, really, thinking it was maybe just something my particular body didn't do. Then, in the spring of my junior year, I mentioned to a (platonic) girlfriend that I'd never reached the big O. And she was like, well, have you tried to give yourself one?

The thing about me and masturbation up until that point was this: I'd kinda done it, but I kinda hadn't. I remember from a young age that it felt good to touch myself "down there." Sometimes, as a kid, I'd linger my fingers there when I wiped myself in the bathroom. I could lose myself in those lovely rubbing sensations long enough that my mother would wonder what was taking me so long. As I grew up, the rubbing moved to the bedroom, but if you'd asked me if I masturbated, I would have said no. It was more of an idle pastime, something I would indulge in when my hand would first brush my labia for more innocent reasons, like putting on underwear or climbing into bed. If that brush felt good and I had time, I'd rub a little while. But I never once thought to myself: *Now I am going to give myself sexual pleasure.* Not because I thought there was anything wrong with doing that, it just literally never occurred to me. No one ever spoke to me about it—as far as I knew, I knew no females who did it. Not until that spring of my junior year, when my friend insisted it was the best thing ever.

That night, I did as she'd suggested. I closed the door to my bedroom, grabbed some oil, and got comfortable. And then I rubbed in a new way, with intention. I explored what types of touch in what places made sensation more or less intense, what rhythms made that intensity build or slowed it. I took my time. I let my mind wander. And then I let it clear as I focused all of my attention on the pleasure expanding from my clitoris. I relaxed into the tension until it felt deliciously unbearable. And then, to my life-changing astonishment, I allowed that swelling pressure to break open and explode and convulse and radiate up through my body until I had gooseflesh and the tip of my nose was tingling.

After that, I never once faked an orgasm ever again. Not only is lying toxic to a relationship, but I don't want to cheat myself out of that experience, or give a lover misleading information about what gets me off. More important, since then, I've always made the time to masturbate, because it's free and it's good for me and it makes me feel great. There aren't enough things in the world you can say all three things about, so I try not to deny myself the ones that I find. This week, I'm going to ask that you don't, either.

Dive In: As you spend this week bringing some healing to the parts of you that feel freaky and undesirable, I want you to affirm the opposite every single day via the act of self-love. Regardless of whether you have other sexual partners, I want you to set aside time

every single day, for the next seven, to give sexual pleasure to yourself, by yourself.

How you do it is up to you. Vibrators, fingers, whatever you prefer. And orgasms don't have to be the point,
but it should feel as explicitly sexual as you can handle.
Maybe you'll think about fantasies or past experiences
that turn you on. Maybe you'll just focus on the physical
sensations. What matters is you, giving yourself sexual
pleasure, every day this week. If you want more in-depth
advice, I highly recommend Betty Dodson's classic book
Sex for One.

If you're already a practiced masturbator, use this week to
explore new approaches, the way Buffy did:

*I've pretty much masturbated the same way and thought
about the same kind of stuff forever. So I took this as an
opportunity to try different methods, and different positions, and different tools and toys, and stuff to break up
the monotony. I've realized after this week that masturbation had become really monotonous for me, almost like
my sex life with myself needed some spicing up. It was
really nice to explore my sexuality in a way I hadn't let
myself before.*

TRIGGER FINGERS

Sometimes masturbation can bring up uncomfortable feelings
or bad memories. Maybe you've internalized the message that
it's wrong, and can't shake that feeling. Maybe you've been

shamed for being sexual, and this reminds you of that feeling. Maybe you've been sexually violated in some way, and this brings back those feelings. Maybe you don't even know why. There's nothing wrong with you if that happens. Sexual pleasure can feel really loaded, depending on our histories, and a lot of that history is lodged in our bodies. You may feel fine just thinking about sexual pleasure, but experiencing it can be a whole different ball of wax, for reasons you may not even understand at first.

These sudden negative responses are often called "triggers," because they can come on suddenly and without much provocation and trigger an overwhelming bad feeling. Here's what author Staci Haines has to say about them in her book, *Healing Sex:*

The idea of embracing your triggers may seem counterintuitive at first. You may feel uncomfortable and unsettled with this way of dealing with triggers, yet I have seen its effectiveness time and time again. Instead of avoiding and moving away from triggers, you can begin to move toward and into them . . . When you move yourself toward and into a trigger, you have the opportunity to then process the material and move through it. In doing this you can release the trigger from your body, emotions, and mind and be complete with it. Triggers act as signposts to what is in need of healing. They guide you on the road to freedom.

Of course, as much as I agree with Haines that you ultimately want to move into a trigger the way you steer into a curve if you're skidding in a car, you'll want to take good care of yourself while you're doing it. You don't have to do it all at once. If you're dealing with triggers, or suspect this daily masturbation may be triggering, try to let supportive friends and/or counselors know that you may need them a little more right now. Make a plan for how best to take care of yourself, whether that's upping the amount of time you spend on nonsexual body love, talking it out with someone, or employing other strategies.

"When I get triggered," says Elizabeth, age forty-one, "I remove myself from the triggering source, then go hold an ice cube in my hand until the sensation of cold redirects my mind. I'll also talk to a friend if there's someone available."

If you find you need more support dealing with your triggers than this brief section can provide, I highly recommend checking out Haines's book, *The Survivors' Guide to Sex,* and/or the classic healing workbook, Ellen Bass's *The Courage to Heal.* Even if you don't identify as a survivor of sexual violence, these books are a treasure trove of information, exploration, and support for those of us for whom sex sometimes feels emotionally painful.

So. Start your engine. Masturbation Week has begun. Thus fortified by self-pleasuring, let's figure out how to deal with your freaky, geeky feelings. The ones that tell you you're too fat, too skinny, too young, too old, too queer, too trans, too dark, too mixed, too poor, too kinky, too foreign, too inexperienced, too damaged, too weak, too aggressive, too depressed, too smart, too stupid, too successful, too much of a failure, too . . . well, too *too* to be desired in any good way.

We're going to help you heal those feelings not just because you deserve healing, but because living in that place can be unhealthy at best, dangerous at worst. As Zeinab puts it:

I was never really desired by anybody in my school, and in college, that sort of continued. And when I go out with my friends, I'm never approached, so in the rare moments when someone does talk to me, there's always this thought in my head: Oh, this person's talking to me. They might find me sexually attractive. *So there have been times when . . . even if I wasn't interested in a person, just the fact that they were interested in me was something that piqued my interest. And I end up doing things that I regret later, because I feel like it's my only chance to experience something sexually.*

MAKING FRIENDS WITH YOUR FEELINGS

Just like our intuition, women's feelings are much maligned. We're assumed to be extremely "emotional," and our voices and opinions are routinely dismissed because of these much-hyped feelings. This often leaves us with a wary and fraught relationship with our own feelings—especially the "negative" ones, like anger and grief and sadness and frustration. On the other hand, we are welcome to have "positive" emotions, because those always seem to benefit others, don't they? We're admonished to "smile" by strangers on the street, expected to be sweet and cheerful in social situations, and encouraged to never let our less-than-happy moods show, lest it bring anybody down. In short, be Mary Poppins or any number of Disney heroines.

Becca, age twenty-six, has struggled with her feelings for years: "I have a stubborn belief that I should be able to think my feelings into other feelings. Like, if I don't like being angry or sad, that if I feel strongly enough about it, I should be able to change it. And that's not true. That's been a lesson I've had to learn over and over again. Willpower isn't enough."

Feelings—even the "bad" ones—can be your friend. They give you key information about what you want more of, and what you've had quite enough of, thank you very much. They can tune you in to moments when you need to focus more on self-care—like when you're cranky and, when you stop to think about it, you realize it's because you haven't eaten all day. They can also guide you out of stuck places you can't "think" your way out of, like a relationship that just doesn't feel right, even though "on paper" everything looks fine.

What's more, there's no cure for them but to feel them. As Winston Churchill once said, "If you're going through hell, keep going." In other words, our tendency is to freeze up and resist when we feel painful feelings. But that's exactly how to keep them around longer. If you want difficult feelings to give way to easier ones, the best way to do that, counterintuitive though it may seem, is to give those challenging emotions the attention they require. (Sound like the advice on triggers earlier? There's a good reason for that.)

So if you're feeling angry/sad/frustrated/self-conscious about being you in all your freaky geekdom, and not someone else for whom sexuality seems a whole lot easier, the first thing to do is just feel that. That feeling is real, and it's yours, but it won't last forever. It sure seems like it will. It feels like if you let yourself start crying, you'll cry forever. Or if you let yourself experience the rage that you've been trying to suppress, you'll smash the whole world in. I've been there. I know. And the only thing that ever helps is taking a leap of faith and letting the feeling come anyhow. Given enough time and expression, the feeling always shifts. It fades or morphs or dissipates or mellows or evolves. It doesn't stay the same.

But *how* do you feel your feelings? How do you feel them in ways that are healing and not hurtful? Here are a few guidelines:

Always Remember That Feelings Aren't Facts

Just because something feels awful doesn't mean it's actually bad for you. For example, the idea of moving in with your partner might feel really scary. That could be because it's not the right thing for you, or it could be because it reminds you of some similar dynamic, like the time you moved in with someone else and later discovered they'd been cheating on you the whole time. Or the time your father left when you were a kid.

Instead of thinking of your feelings as fact, think of them as clues that can lead you to something important to know about yourself. Just the same way that physical sensations can mean any number of things—dangerous drugs can make you feel great in the short term, and having a broken bone reset so it can heal can be excruciatingly painful—so can your emotions. Anger can mean that someone has violated your trust, or it can mean that you're with someone you trust deeply enough that you feel free to experience the full power of your emotions with them. The crucial thing is to pay attention, and to do your best to sort out what your feelings are trying to tell you.

Don't Indulge Feelings About Your Feelings

If you're heartbroken that someone you love left you, it's easy to get so caught up feeling angry at yourself for having trusted them that you don't give yourself space to just feel the heartbreak and grieve for the relationship. That's a perfect recipe for staying stuck. If you want to move through your feelings, the first thing to do is accept that they exist. Say to yourself, "I'm feeling heartbroken right now. I accept that." As they say in *Star Trek:* Resistance is futile.

Reach Out

It's easy to let our difficult feelings isolate us. We fear we'll be judged or misunderstood if we express them to someone. But isolation can make painful emotions fester and mutate and grow. Using your intuition, as well as what you consciously know about your friends and family, pick one or two confidants who you have good reason to believe will handle your feelings with care, and then ask if they're willing to talk. The goal here isn't to come up with solutions, it's to express your feelings and have them witnessed by someone else. That simple act can make them feel more manageable and help you feel less alone. If you can't find anyone close to you to talk with, try Befrienders.org— the site will help you find a hotline in your area where you can reach volunteers trained to listen to difficult emotions.

Remember That Actions Have Consequences

It's fine (and sometimes awesome!) to let your feelings motivate you to act, but emotions aren't a get-out-of-jail-free card, either literally or figuratively. If you lash out at someone, they're probably going to be hurt or angry or both. If you are physically violent to yourself or someone else, there may be real medical or legal consequences. If you blow off work because you don't feel up to getting out of bed, you may get reprimanded or fired.

There's Nothing Wrong with "Being Emotional"

This is a hard one to undo, because you've probably been taught the opposite over and over. You know, crying is a sign of weakness, angry women are strident harpies, outspoken women are bitchy. Whatever the stereotype, most of us have been dismissed (or threatened with dismissal) because of our feelings. But your feelings can be a superpower! Knowing and embracing them can give you clarity like nothing else, and that's the kind of clarity that can get you to what you really really want, both in sex and in life in general. After all, you can't express your desires or boundaries until you know what they feel like. Think of feelings like a spigot in a sink: There's just one on/off valve. If you close off anger, you're closing off your ability to feel joy and satisfaction and pleasure, too. Instead, open the spigot a little at a time, and learn to manage the flow. The energy of your emotions can be like a power plant for your whole life.

Dive In: Meditation is a really fantastic way to make friends with your feelings. Try this very simple practice: In a quiet place, sit upright (if you can) in a comfortable but engaged position. For many people, that's with their legs crossed, possibly with a pillow under their butt. Or invent your own position. Be sure to do what you need to support your position so that it's as close to pain-free as possible. Now close your eyes and breathe deeply, slowly, through your nose. Focus on your breath. Feel the air come in, feel it release. Over and over. If thoughts or feelings arise, notice them, but don't attach. Imagine that they're clouds floating through the sky. Don't worry about what the clouds mean. They're clouds. Don't worry if they'll stay or go or change—you know they'll morph and eventually disappear. Try doing this for ten minutes, and then whenever you notice yourself becoming overwhelmed by or struggling against your emotions.

And if your feelings themselves are what make you feel like a freak, well, you're not alone.

STRONG IN THE BROKEN PLACES

If you think of yourself as a little different or off-kilter in ways that relate to your sexuality, or at least your ability to be sexual with a partner, you are not alone. I don't think I know a single woman who doesn't feel that way. Whether you've got a mental illness like anxiety or depression that affects your libido or your ability to deal with people, or you have a history of sexual trauma, or an eating disorder, or an addiction, or your history has taught you some twisted things about sex and relationships, or even if you have suffered more than your fair share of heartbreak and it's left you twitchy and mistrustful, it's easy to convince yourself you're too "damaged" to find satisfying sexual partners. That no one will want to do the work required to be with you, because they could be with any number of infinitely "simpler" women.

Whatever the case, it's important not to confuse this feeling with truth, and I'll tell you why:

Everybody Has Issues

No, seriously. Even that perfect-seeming woman your ex left you for, with the perfect hair and the perfect life and the perfect friends and the perfect career saving puppies from certain death. I'll tell you a secret about her: She's not perfect. When you compare your insides to someone's outsides, it's never a fair fight. In other words, we all try to present our best self to the world. I'm amazed sometimes by the people who think I have it all together. Because, boy howdy, if you spent a few days as a fly on my wall, you'd know differently. I'm not even going to tell you what you'd see, because I'm afraid you'd judge me for it. Which is the point. So when you imagine there are all of those "simple" people out there who are so much less messed up than you, it's at least 50 percent bunk. Some people are just better at hiding their messes than others. And sometimes the folks who hide them well are the most messed-up in the end.

Even so, maybe you have more "issues" than the average woman. That's possible—if there's a bell curve of "messed up," some of us have got to be on the more-messed-up tail of it. Let's say for the sake of argument that you are. Well, your potential partners will be different, too. I'm not saying that you should look for someone with similar issues, because it's hard to even make those equations anyhow. But just like there are people out there attracted to women of all shapes and sizes, there are also people out there who find the "simpler" or so-called "normal" people a little boring or unchallenging but really spark with people who are more complicated, or who've lived a little more, or who've had to face challenges and learn how to deal with the real world.

If you've got challenging issues, it may make getting what you really really want harder, because you've got extra feelings to manage for yourself and extra needs and boundaries to negotiate with your partners. And you may require greater levels of trust with a partner than the "less messed-up" people do, because you may want to have some clue they can handle what you're dealing with before you get down with them.

On the other hand, the skills you're learning in order to manage whatever your particular issues are can also be an asset in sexual connections. In *A Farewell to Arms,* Ernest Hemingway wrote, "The world breaks every one and afterward many are strong at the broken places." Odds are, that describes you in more ways that you know. The places where we're broken are often places we've developed special muscles. Sometimes those muscles are literal—if your legs are weak, you may have developed strong arms to help you get around, and those strong arms can be a real asset when it comes to holding a lover close. (And they may be a turn-on to a girl like me, who has a preference for strong shoulders.) Sometimes your arms are stronger metaphorically—you've had to develop really great communication skills in order to stick up for yourself around whatever makes you feel freaky, and those communication skills can be put to great use in the sack. Or you've developed a strong empathy for other freaky people, and that helps potential partners feel safe with you. Maybe dealing with obstacles has forced you to become more creative, and that makes you a more creative lover.

Becca knows both sides of this:

My transgender identity has definitely impacted both my sexual experiences and how I think about sex. On the frustrating end, it's meant I've been bombarded with messages about the "abnormality" of my body and my desire to be sexual: chicks with dicks, she-males, and the like. On the other hand, being trans has given me the opportunity to think lots more about my gender and sexual expression than I think most folks do. And it's left me very in touch with my desires, both for my physicality and for sexual interaction. I'm still working on communicating those desires, but I think even simply acknowledging them is a big step in the right direction.

In the end, it's important to make room for both truths: There are things about you that make life harder that you can't change. And dealing with those things, navigating through a world that discriminates against you because of them, has given you skills and powers that people who have it "easier" may never attain.

Dive In: Get a large piece of paper or even poster board. On it, write in big, bold letters a word or words that describe the ways you feel "freaky." Get real: Use the words that stir up the strongest feelings in you, both positively and negatively (fat, loud, ugly, badass, weak, dark, shy, gross, etc.). Add images, colors, symbols—whatever ways you want to represent the parts of you that feel undesirable or "other." Take your time. Make it feel as complete as you can.

When it feels done, sit down and just look at it for a while. Feel your feelings. Don't try to control them, but don't act on them right now, either. Just feel them. Notice them. Welcome them.

Next, write for ten minutes about the ways the qualities or circumstances you've represented on your poster have made sexuality harder for you. Don't try to play anything down. Nothing is too minor or major here.

Now, if you can, get out a candle, place it in front of your poster, and light it. As you watch the flame, allow yourself to grieve for the opportunities for pleasure you've lost or never had, because of the way the world treats your "difference." Let yourself feel loss, or anger, or helplessness, or whatever you feel. Do this for as long as you like, for at least ten minutes. Resist the impulse to try to cheer yourself up. But welcome acceptance of your feelings and circumstances if it comes.

When you're ready, get out your notebook again and write for ten minutes about the skills and powers you've developed to help negotiate your "difference" in the world, and how you do or could apply those powers to your sexual interactions. Ignore any voices in your head telling you it won't work. Be creative. Be hopeful. Be idealistic.

When you're done with that, blow out the candle, but leave the poster up somewhere where you'll see it every day for a week. Notice your feelings every time you look at it. Try not to judge or change your feelings—whatever they are, they're the right ones.

At the end of the week, you can do whatever you want with the poster. Burn it. Drown it. Chop it to bits. Fold it away somewhere so you can take it out and look at it when you want. Leave it up as a powerful reclamation of your freakiness. Hang it in a museum. It's entirely up to you.

THE WRONG REASONS

Sometimes the issue isn't whether someone wants you or not. It's whether or not they want you for the right reasons. Which begs the question: What are reasons you want to be desired sexually, and what are reasons that make you feel bad?

It's not a trick question. For some people, it goes back to the conversation about love that we started in the last chapter. If you want to have sex only in the context of a love relationship, then "you turn me on" is a wrong reason to be wanted. "I love you and I think you're beautiful inside and out" is probably a right reason. On the other hand, if you're not looking for anything serious, "I want to cherish every inch of you, and only you, till death do us part" can be a totally wrong reason to be desired, but "you are so incredibly hot" might be a great one. It all depends on what you really really want.

But there's a deeper, more twisted kind of Wrong Reason, which has everything to do with feeling like a freak. Whether

it's our big butts, our dark skin, our queer or transgender iden-
tity/body, our age, or any number of things, many of us have
had experiences with people who made us feel like even less
than the sum of our parts. Some people call this "fetishizing,"
some others call it "othering" or "objectifying," but whatever
you call it, it can feel really bad. Like you're no longer a person,
you're just whatever the "freaky" or "different" part of you
symbolizes to the person who wants you.

Don't get me wrong—we all have tastes. Some of us like
curvier, plusher bodies, and some like firmer ones. Some are
more drawn to creamy skin, and some to caramel. As I mentioned earlier, I'm a sucker for strong shoulders. There's nothing wrong with having preferences. But I've had plenty of lovers with average-to-weak shoulders, because shoulders aren't
the only thing I care about. Where it veers into Wrong Reason
territory is when a partner is so focused on a particular preference that we feel reduced to that one quality. And it's especially charged when that quality is something that has been used
to take power away from us, something that has made us feel
weird or different or "other" throughout our lives, like our race
or our sexual orientation.

What's especially insidious about this fetishizing kind of
Wrong Reason is that it can become a generalized fear that no
one will ever want you as a whole person. And when that happens, you can easily wind up closing yourself off to people who
may want you for completely awesome reasons, because you're
afraid of encountering the Wrong Reasons.

For Zeinab, that means:

When I think about approaching someone, I'm always second-guessing myself because I'm basically at the bottom when it comes to racial hierarchies in this country. So why should I even bother talking with someone when I feel like the chances of them being interested in the real me are slim to none? And if they are interested in me, is it because of a legitimate reason?

There are no easy solutions here, but there are a few ways to help you sort out whether someone wants you for you, or for something you symbolize to them. Depending on how well you know them, you could just ask. But there's always the chance that they may not be aware they're treating you like a symbol. It may be completely unintentional, and you may or may not be able to help them see it. (And you may or may not be willing to put in the effort required to try.) What matters is how it feels to you: Do you feel like you get to be a whole, complex person with them? Or do you feel boxed in, stereotyped, or extra-freaky? If it's any of the latter qualities, and you either can't or don't want to work through it with the person, it may be time to move on. Because choosing to stay with someone who makes you feel bad about yourself—even if they don't mean to—is sending yourself the message that you deserve to feel bad about yourself.

On the flip side, try to notice those lovers or potential lovers who are attracted to more than one thing about you. Sure, maybe your queerness is a turn-on for them, but so are your laugh and your hazel eyes. As you spend more time together and reveal different sides of yourself, are they more attracted, or are they trying to shove you back into the box they think you belong in? Don't get hung up on whether or not they're hot for some part of you that makes you feel freaky—pay attention to whether or not that's the *only* part they're into, or the biggest part.

As fat activist Brian Stuart puts it (he's talking about love, not sexual attraction, here, but the point remains the same):

Our culture creates a false choice between being loved for something and being loved in spite of it. Loving someone for a trait is often framed as a negative, especially fat, while the other is exalted as a virtue. But why is loving someone "in spite of" who they are at all honorable? That's not a good thing. It's about enforcing cultural standards, not true love.

I figure there are two less objectionable variants of these standards. You can love someone with genuinely no regard to something so it's not something you are explicitly martyring yourself over, as in the "in spite of" construction. Or you can love someone inclusive of, where there is a genuine attraction to a specific trait but that is not the entirety of the attraction.

Dive In: Take out your timeline, and add in times when you've felt like a symbol or fetish object to someone else. Then pick one of those incidents and write about it. What was it that the person did or said that inspired those feelings? Do you think they knew they were making you feel that way? Do you think they cared? How did you handle the situation? How do you wish you'd handled it? How do you think you'd handle it if it happened today?

GET INTO THE DRIVER'S SEAT

In the end, the number one best way to stop worrying that no one will want you, or no one will want you for the right reasons, is to stop thinking of yourself as an abandoned pet in a rescue shelter, waiting for someone to pick you, and start thinking of yourself as a whole person who gets to do picking of her own. In other words: Instead of wondering if one trait or another of yours will prevent anyone from wanting to be with you, start focusing on what traits *you* want in a lover.

For some of us, this is obvious. For others, it's a daunting task, because we've never let ourselves entertain such an idea before. For still others, it feels dangerous, because being sexually proactive—being the choos*er* as opposed to the chosen—is something we've learned we're never supposed to do. But now you know how to manage your feelings if they come up, so go ahead and do that, and let's proceed.

There are a lot of ways to approach this question, some of which have to do with the work you did in the last chapter. If you're searching primarily for a long-term, monogamous life partner, you'll probably have different criteria than someone who's looking for a reliable friend with benefits. But in general, there are four categories to think about when considering what makes a good lover for you:

Appearance

It's okay to get a little superficial! Physical attraction matters, and you're allowed to be choosy. Do you find yourself drawn to strong shoulders, soft curves, or striking eyes? What kind of posterior is your preference? Gender factors in here, too: Some of us are attracted more to masculinity, some to femininity, some to androgyny or genderqueerness. It's all okay. You'll probably find that the more deep and lasting a partner you're looking for, the less this will matter, but you don't have to pretend you don't care!

Character

What is the person you're looking for like on the inside? What principles (if any!) guide their behavior? And do they actually act according to these principles, or do they merely talk a good game and behave otherwise? This category includes things like honesty and loyalty, but also religious and political beliefs, and social attitudes, too.

Circumstances

Does your ideal partner have a job? What kind of lifestyle do they lead? How much money do they make? Do they live close by or far away? The circumstances in which someone lives their life can really impact a relationship, and you get to decide which ones are ideal for you, which ones you can work with, and which ones just won't fly.

Skills and Talents

We all get dealt a different hand when it comes to what we're capable of, and we all need partners who contribute different things. Is it important that your sexual partners are funny? Smart? Good dancers? Sweet with children? Great at communication? This is where you can get specific about bedroom skills, too: How talented does your partner need to be in the sack, and what qualifies as sexual talent to you?

Once you figure out what qualities you want in a partner, it's time to add another layer of choosiness: How important is each quality to you? Because, let's get real, nobody's perfect, and you're unlikely to find someone who simultaneously checks all of your boxes. Maybe you'd love to have a partner who is really athletic, but you wouldn't rule out someone who was less active. On the other hand, it may be a total deal breaker if your partner doesn't like to read. Get clear on what's cake vs. what's icing, and you'll be steering yourself toward what you really really want before you know it.

Dive In: Make a list of all the characteristics your ideal partner would have. Be sure to list at least five things in each of the four major categories above. Now, mark each of those characteristics with a "1" if it's a must-have, top-tier, deal-breaker kind of priority; a "2" if it's pretty important but you'd be willing to compromise on it if most of the other important stuff were in place; and a "3" if that characteristic would be nice to have in a sexual partner but hardly is mandatory.

Now, think about your last few sexual partners (or even just people you've been seriously attracted to). How do they measure up? Did you get with them (or want to) because they're what you really really want, or for some other reason (like, they wanted you and you didn't feel like you could pass up the opportunity)?

Don't expect your lists to stay set in stone. Many factors can change them, so it's a good idea to redo them every so often. Prerna learned that through experience.

I'm currently in a long-distance relationship. If you had asked me before if I would ever purposely choose to be in a long-distance relationship, I don't think I would have said yes. And if it was anyone else, I probably wouldn't say yes. But because of this specific relationship, and this specific person, I was able to make where he lives be a three, whereas if you'd asked me several months ago, it would've been a one. I was able to move that down on the list because of how high his other qualities are on my list.

 Go Deeper:

1. Write an ad for yourself. Not a personal ad designed to "sell" you to a prospective partner, but an ad that focuses on what's really great about you. Ads too often are demeaning to women, concentrating on features such as

appearance and sexual invitation, but they don't have to be. This gives you an important challenge: to think through what you have to offer the world out there.

So start by listing all the things that make you a great person. Maybe you are loyal or funny. Maybe you make a great lasagna. You're a good listener. Your lips are really cute and expressive. Build your ad from there, and list every little thing that is cool about you. You know yourself better than anyone, but if you need help, feel free to ask trusted friends to help design your ad.

(Bonus points if you're single and you'd like to meet someone for sex and/or a relationship, but you've been reluctant to put yourself out there: Once you've finished your ad, go ahead and turn it into a real one on an online dating site! This isn't an ad to attract someone who might "pick" you; it's a way to expand your choices and make it possible to do picking of your own. Don't stop until you've completed every field, even if you have to ask a friend for help. Remember, you don't have to say yes to anyone just because they email you (or even if you email them and change your mind). Just create some new options for yourself, and take notice of how the process feels. Do you feel afraid? Of what? Do a risk assessment on that fear, using the tools we learned in chapter 4.)

2. Every product comes with a care manual. Write one. What things make you keep going, and keep you happy and satisfied? What instructions can

you give yourself for daily maintenance, or an
annual service? Go wild, and shoot for the stars—
from bubble baths to long hikes, from credit for
your accomplishments to phone calls with friends
to, yes, even sexual pleasure, list all the things that
make you happy and contented.

3. Create a new you. Ever wish you could try out
    life from inside someone else's skin? If you have
    access to an Internet connection, you can. Visit an
    alternate-reality digital world like *The Sims* (www
    .wyrrw.com/sims) or *Second Life*[1] (www.wyrrw.com/
    secondlife), and create an avatar (that's a digital
    representation of you) that you think looks both
    powerful and desirable. Now, try interacting with
    other avatars in that world. If you feel up to it, try
    out some behaviors that are outside of your com-
    fort zone—flirt openly if you're usually too shy; set
    forceful boundaries if that doesn't come easily to
    you in "real life." Play. See how it feels. How much
    do you feel like a different person, and how much
    do you still feel like you? How do people respond
    to you, and how does that match up with how you
    expect them to respond?

CHAPTER 7

LET'S TALK
ABOUT SEX, BABY

B E VEWWWY QUIET. WE'RE HUNTING WAAAAAABIT.
Those of you who are familiar with the Bugs Bunny oeu-
vre know that this was the strategy of one Elmer Fudd, wabbit
hunter. And you'll also know how well that code of silence
tended to work out for him (hint: not that well). And yet we
so often try the same disastrous strategy when it comes to sex.

The silence around sex works differently depending on
your gender. For women, we're of course not supposed to have
any of our own sexual desires, and if we do, heaven forbid
that we pursue them in any active way. And even if we do, it's
supposed to be through dressing sexy, making ourselves seem
ultra-available, twirling our hair coquettishly. Under no circumstances are we supposed to speak out loud, and with intent,
about our desire—or anything having to do with it. That would
make us sluts, and you know what happens to them.

Men don't get off any easier when it comes to sex talk, of
course. Our culture teaches them that they're supposed to be

conquering their partners, not communicating with them. So they're often left feeling that they're supposed to psychically know what their partners want better than their partners even do, all without uttering a word. A guy who has to ask is hardly a man, you know.

I'm sure you can imagine what I think of this whole setup. But it's more than bunk: It's dangerous. Imposed silence around sex and sexuality keeps us alienated from what we really really want, and it also gives rise to the kinds of misunderstandings that can do real emotional and physical damage. So take a deep breath, because we're going to take Salt-N-Pepa's advice: Let's talk about sex.

The first person you need to learn how to communicate with about sex is yourself. Seems silly on some level, but it's no less true: If you can't admit to yourself what you want and don't want when it comes to sex, you're in no condition to share that information with anyone else. Of course, that's a big part of what this whole book is about—getting real with yourself about your own desires and boundaries. So give yourself a little pat on the back. You're already on your way. But just for kicks, let's take a moment now and practice specifics.

Dive In: Every day this week, in your daily writing, write about one thing you want or don't want when it comes to sex. Be as specific as you can: "I want to have my hair pulled" is good, as is "I don't want to ever try anal sex." Practice now. Make a list of five things you definitely do or don't want when it comes to sex.

It can be scary to admit, even to ourselves, what we really really want. Vague desires seem so much more real when we put them into words. But don't worry. Just because you wrote down that you really really want to cover your partner in chocolate syrup, it doesn't mean you have to do it. Go back to that list of five things, and put stars next to any things on that list that you want to do but don't want to do for real right now. Everybody's got desires they're not ready (and may never be ready) to act on. Communicating with yourself about those kinds of boundaries is just as important as being honest about the things you want (or don't want) right now.

Of course, if you're going to be sexual with someone else, you're going to have to sort out how to communicate what you really really want with them, too. And that can be twice as tricky, since, even if you feel comfortable being straight-up about your sexual needs, your lover may not be comfortable hearing about them yet, or sharing their own desires. That can be hard. In an ideal world, we would have sexual partners who already feel good about direct communication. But sometimes partners like that are hard to find, and sometimes we're already in love (or in lust!) with someone before we find out they're hung up on how to get the words out. So we may have to help them along, even as we're struggling ourselves. That's okay. Life is messy sometimes, and so is sex.

DO I HAVE TO?

Let's start by talking about why to communicate directly. How many times have you said or heard some version of this:

"I don't know. One minute we were dancing, and then the next thing I knew we had just had sex. It kind of just happened."

"We woke up together, and she was like, 'So, when can I see you again?' And now I guess we're in a relationship? It just happened."

"It just happened" is incredibly common when it comes to sexual relationships. It's also the enemy of what you really really want.

When we say "it just happened" (and we don't mean "I was incredibly drunk or high or asleep and therefore not aware enough of my surroundings to have actively participated," which is sexual assault, not sex), what we're doing is denying responsibility for our sexual and romantic decisions. That can feel pretty appealing, especially if you're not comfortable with your sexuality or don't believe you deserve pleasure and safety. If we imagine that sex and relationships "just happen" to us, that they're really beyond our control, then we can't be blamed for anything that goes wrong, or shamed for being the sexual people we are, or feel embarrassed for wanting satisfaction.

Trouble is, "it just happened" also denies us the opportunity to be active in pursuit of our own pleasure. There's no room in "it just happened" to know what you really really want, so there can't be any room to pursue it.

Letting things "just happen" can also be risky. If you're refusing responsibility for decision making, you're also probably paying less attention to your intuition. And you're less likely to speak up if something feels off, or if you want your partner to practice safer sex, or if something starts to hurt or freak you out and you want to stop.

It's not even always high-stakes negotiations where this winds up mattering. Take pity sex, for example. I slept with a guy out of pity once. It was horrible. We were on a first date, and he was funny and charming and smart and handsome, and basically let him know I was interested in sleeping with him before we even kissed. (Please take my advice and never do this: The way someone kisses can tell you a lot about how they'll do other things.) So we went back to his room, and as we're leaning in for that first kiss, he makes a stiff "O" with his lips and pokes his tongue out of it—before our lips even touch. I can still see it, coming at me in slow motion, and in my brain a thought flashed up as though on a screen: *I've made a serious miscalculation. Abort! Abort!*

But did I? No, I felt too bad. It felt too impossibly awkward for me to stop him midkiss and say, "Actually, I've changed my mind." So I slept with him. And it was terrible. I was just checked out the whole time, wondering when it would be over, and he was like an overenthusiastic, unhousebroken puppy. He had no idea how miserable I was, but that wasn't his fault—I was actively lying. Through my actions and my affect, I was doing my best to convince him I was having a great time, too.

Did anything horrible happen? Unless you count the hives I had at the end of the evening (his dog? His scratchy wool blanket? I still don't know), not really. I felt icky about it for a day or two (and still do when I think about it, including now), and I had to awkwardly tell him I just wasn't that into him when he followed up for a second date. Which must've been confusing for him, since I'd given him no sign the night before that I wasn't into him.

But it was also confusing for me, in dangerous ways—
the same ways it's always confusing and dangerous when you
ignore your instincts and violate your own boundaries. Which is
why, if I ever find myself in a similar situation again, I hope my
emotional muscles will be strong enough to allow me to speak
up sooner.

It can be really tempting to leave these decisions up to other
people. When you let someone else lead, you're not required to
put yourself out there as much. If rejection feels scary to you,
that can be awfully appealing. You can also avoid rejecting
other people by going with their flow, at least in the short term.
(Though trust that I speak from experience when I tell you that
not telling someone you're not that into them when you're not
that into them only leads to bad things for both of you down
the road.)

But here's the thing: You can't have sexual relationships
without messy, awkward, emotionally risky interactions. You
just can't. You can deal with the messy, awkward, emotionally
risky stuff up front and honestly and increase your chances of
having fulfilling mutual interactions, or you can wait and hope
it doesn't blow up in your face. But you can't engage on such an
intimate level with another human being without it sometimes
being weird. The sooner you make peace with that and stop
imagining this stuff is easy for everyone but you (because it's
not: It's messy, risky, and emotionally awkward for everyone),
the sooner you'll stop letting things "just happen" and take control of your sexual and romantic life.

And the sooner you do that, the sooner you'll discover how
awesome it can be. Talking freely about sex and safety with your

partners not only makes sex more fun and relaxed—because you're worrying less and getting more of what you really really want—but also makes it easier to tell the great partners from the ones you want to avoid before you get too hurt. And that information means your intuition will get better and better, which means you'll get even better at knowing your own desires and boundaries and finding people who can simultaneously respect and satisfy you. In short: It's the best possible kind of positive-feedback loop.

Dive In: Pay attention this week to the times when you're not speaking up. Do you want seconds at dinner but are afraid to say so? Do you actually want to wear that outfit, or are you doing it because you think someone else will like it on you? Did your friend or partner hurt your feelings, but you aren't letting them know? Make a note each time it happens. Then, when you've got some time, pick one example and write about what it felt like. And then write about what it might have felt like if you had gone the other way and spoken on your own behalf.

WHAT TO SAY AND WHEN TO SAY IT

There are five basic things you'll ideally want to communicate about with any new sexual partner. They are:

- *Turn-ons and turnoffs.* This may seem obvious, but if you don't tell your partner what gets your motor running and what makes you stall out, you're a lot less likely to get the good stuff. Plus, assuming

you're having sex with a decent person, your partner
probably will be quite relieved to get some guidance.

- *Your STD status.* Do you have a sexually transmitted
  disease? Does your partner? How sure are you both?
  How recently have you been tested? What were you
  each tested for? What risks have you encountered
  since you were last tested?

- *Safer sex practices.* What's required to bring the disease and pregnancy risks of sex to a level you each
  feel comfortable with? Can you both commit to
  doing what's required?

- *Consent and boundaries.* What kinds of activities can
  you both enthusiastically consent to, and what happens when you want to say no?

- *Expectations.* Is this a no-strings-attached hookup?
  The beginning of a life together? Something in
  between, or something else entirely? The sooner
  you're clear with each other about it, the better you'll be at avoiding hurting each other
  unnecessarily.

This may sound like a lot of chitchat to get through before
you get naked, but it doesn't have to be. (And it doesn't have to
be finished before you take your clothes off.) As you get more
comfortable with these conversations, you'll find that they can
be brief, easy exchanges, at least when you're with partners who
care about your needs. Some, like the STD status and safer sex
talks, can be quickly dispatched, and others, like your turn-ons
and turnoffs, can be ongoing conversations that unspool both
in and out of bed. You'll get the hang of it, I promise. The

important thing is to just open your mouth and start. Which brings us to . . .

If You Can't Get the Words Out.

Let's get real for a minute: All this communication stuff may seem simple on paper, but it's a lot harder to do in practice, isn't it? When it comes to talking about sex with our partners, many of us are woefully short on practice. That's not our fault (for reasons we've already explored in this chapter), but it can still be a real obstacle, like it was for Ruby, age twenty:

> *Because my "hookups" had always happened when my partner and I were drunk, the first time I hooked up with someone soberly I realized I had never advocated for myself sexually before. In fact, I didn't even find I had the language to advocate for myself. When I think back on this hookup, I realize I let a lot of things happen that I wasn't comfortable with. And I always used to think, I'm an outspoken feminist; I don't get taken advantage of, but I felt completely silenced.*

So what to do when you want to have a key sex talk but can't seem to get the words out? There are no magic solutions, but there are a few approaches that can help.

Use Your Strengths

I could write a little Mad Libs–style script here to help you learn how to communicate with your partner(s) about sex. I thought about doing that. But no matter what I write, some of you would look at it and think, *Are you kidding me? She wants me to say what? No way would I ever say that.*

And you'd be right. We all have our own strengths when it comes to communication. Some of us rely on humor when we want to get something across. Some of us are frank, unable to resist the direct approach. Some of us prefer talking things through in person, while others would rather have a personal conversation via email or phone.

What's important is to know your style and, if possible, the style preferences of your partner. Consider tone (blunt, sincere, funny, etc.), time (ASAP vs. need-some-time-to-think), and method of delivery (in person, phone, email, IM, text message, smoke signal, whatever). For example, I'm a pretty direct gal. I like to say what's on my mind as clearly and simply as possible. But I was in a relationship for a long while with a guy who would feel really cornered by my blunt declarations. Eventually we figured out that he found it much easier to deal when I sent them via email so he had time to think and feel and work out his response, and didn't feel so much like he was in the hot seat. While I prefer to communicate in person, that's much less important to me than being able to communicate directly, so I was happy to roll with that.

You may not know your sexual communication style yet, but I bet you know a thing or two about what approaches you gravitate toward when you're feeling awkward or vulnerable. Of course, context matters too—if you'd rather talk things out on the phone in advance, it's going to make spontaneous hook-ups harder to navigate. In cases like that, you've got a choice to make: Would you rather learn a new skill or choose different kinds of sexual interactions?

> ~~~ **Dive In:** Ask three trusted friends about your communication style. Ask them to think of a time the two of you talked about something uncomfortable or difficult, and ask them what they remember about the approach you took. Take notes on what they say. Do they all agree? Are you different with different people? Do you agree with their impressions?

Tell on Yourself

It may be that, no matter what approach you try, you can't bring yourself to say, "Can we talk about using condoms?" or, "I like it so much better if it's nice and slow." If you're truly tongue-tied, try telling on yourself. Instead of waiting and waiting until you can blurt out the subject at hand, get there earlier by starting once-removed, saying something like, "I keep wanting to talk with you about something, but it makes me feel so weird." Or whatever describes how you're feeling. That gives your partner a chance to reassure and encourage you before you get to the bit that's tripping you up—and it significantly increases the chances you'll find a way to spit it out sooner rather than later.

Boost Your Confidence

A recent study showed that people who took on the role of a powerful character in a video game for just ninety seconds were more likely to flirt with someone they found attractive afterward than were the folks who didn't play the game.¹ There's a lesson to be learned here, and it's not just about flirting and video games: Doing something that makes us feel confident makes us, well, feel confident. So if you're anxious about sexual communication, one way to work up the nerve is to make sure to do things beforehand that are likely to give you a shot of power. Maybe you're a great cook and you know you can turn out a fantastic dinner. Maybe you're a strong athlete and you want to get a killer workout in. We all have things that make us feel capable and awesome. If you think you may need to do some challenging sexual chatting, find ways to work some confidence-boosters into the hours leading up to it.

As Heidi points out, even just reminding yourself of past accomplishments can work: "No matter what I'm scared to do I think, *Okay, Heidi, you got rid of everything you own, you put everything in a car to move cross-country to live with someone you've never met, you can go to a fucking club.* And that helps."

Dive In: Make a list of things you're great at. Things that make you feel powerful, or at least super-competent. List at least ten things.

Now, identify something you're nervous about this week, whether it's a big meeting at work or a first date. If you haven't got anything to be nervous about this week, congratulations! But also: Pick something that makes you nervous and do it. (Those of you who are shy about flirting with people you're attracted to or asking people out, this is a great opportunity to do just that. Grab a friend and go out to a club or event where there are likely to be people you'll be interested in, or take the plunge and email that person you've had your eye on via an online dating site.) Whatever you choose to do, before you face your fears, do something from your confidence list, even for just a little while.

Do It Anyway

One of the most powerful lessons I took away from both learning and teaching self-defense is this: You can be afraid and be strong at the same time. You can be afraid and do it (whatever "it" is that you know you need to do but scares you) anyway.

We've spent a good deal of time in this book talking about rejecting fear. And that's an awesome goal. But in reality, it doesn't always come easy. Unlearning fear can take a long time, and some fears just never go away. If you wait until you're not afraid, that day may never come, or it may come too late. One of the best gifts you can give yourself is to learn that fear doesn't have to mean freezing. Remember what we discussed about how feelings aren't facts? Well, this is a great example. You can feel your fear and act anyway, like Mag did:

I'm very very afraid of letting people know how vulnerable I am. I'm worried they'll either be disgusted or take advantage, so I try to pass off my emotions with self-deprecating humor. Recently, I was trying to build up my

courage to grab someone's hand, but was too scared and
proud to outright do it. I had to tell on myself and say,
"I'm building up my courage to do something very dorky.
Hold on a moment." Then I took a deep breath and did it.
We held hands the rest of the night, and the next morning
he reached out and took my hand. I felt dazed but happy,
and proud that I did something about how I felt.

Dive In: Write a letter to your fear. Give it a
name if you want, or even draw a picture of it. Then write it
a letter telling it that you're in charge now. Tell it that you'll
listen to it, you'll consider what it has to say, but ultimately,
you're going to do what you need and want to do, and it
can come along if it wants, but it can't stop you. Don't worry
if you believe yourself or not. Write it as if you believe it.

Practice, Practice, Practice

Ultimately, there's no way to get better at sexual communication without doing it. Think of it as a muscle that will get stronger only if you use it—it's going to hurt at first. It may feel sore afterward. If you don't do it regularly, you may not see much of a result (or at least it will take a very long time to see the results you want). On the other hand, if you start small, warm up, and gradually, regularly work your way up, you'll find that things that used to seem impossible are now second nature. Whether it's making sure you talk about STDs or confessing a private fantasy, it will all come more easily the more often you do it.

≈≈ **Dive In:** This is the first of a series of practice conversations I'll be asking you to have this week. For each of them, choose the option that works best for you:

- Have the conversation with an actual partner or friend—whomever you want to have the conversation with for real.

- Ask a friend to role-play the conversation with you in person. Tell them how you want the person they're playing (whether a hypothetical partner or a real, specific person) to respond, or leave it up to them.

- Ask a friend to role-play the conversation with you using technology: You could both have your avatar in *Second Life* or *The Sims* have the conversation, or you could have it over Skype, or chat, or the phone—pick one that feels best to you.

- Play the conversation out yourself in your notebook, writing both parts, one with your left hand, the other with your right.

For this exercise, practice talking with a friend about sex. Pick something you might not normally confide in a friend about, and try it out. How does it feel to say these things out loud? How does your friend respond, and how do those responses feel? Try to pick someone you trust to respond respectfully.

Now that you're ready to get your mouth moving (I meant for talking! Well, and for other stuff, too . . .), let's get specific about the subject matter you'll want to cover.

ENTHUSIASTIC CONSENT

Enthusiastic consent is a simple but crucial principle. What it means is this: It's your partner's responsibility to ensure that you're not just "not objecting" to what's happening between you, sexually speaking, that you're not just allowing whatever's happening to happen. Instead, your partner has to ensure that you're actively enjoying what's going down between the two (or more) of you. And this is equally important: You have the same responsibility to your partner.

Why is enthusiastic consent important? Well, for one, it ensures that everyone's having a good time, and isn't that a good thing? Beyond that, it does several important things:

- It gets past our common cultural assumptions that women are responsible for saying no, and if we don't, or don't do it loudly or repeatedly enough, whatever happens is "our fault." Enthusiastic consent creates a standard where only "yes!" means yes.

- It encourages us to be in ongoing communication with our partners, which fosters playfulness, trust, connection, and dirty talk. (We'll get to dirty talk more in a little bit.)

- It allows us to let go of worry that we might be crossing a line with our partners and instead just relax and enjoy the sex we're having.

There are two tricky parts to enthusiastic consent. One is that it's not always obvious. We can't always tell if our partners are psyched about what we're doing together, for all kinds of reasons. Some people are just more expressive than others, for one. But also, as women, we're often afraid to admit how much we're into sex (there's that slut-shaming fear again), so we act shyer about it than we actually feel. Add in the extra vulnerability that comes from being fully expressive with a partner, and you get to the first subrule of enthusiastic consent: If you can't tell, you have to ask.

What does that mean, exactly? Well, it means that if you're unsure whether your partner is into what you're doing, you just check in. You ask, "Do you like that?" or, "How's this feel, baby?" or any number of other questions that boil down to: Are you into this?

Which brings me to enthusiastic consent subrule number two: Consent is not a light switch. Contrary to what seems like popular belief, sexual consent isn't as simple as "on" or "off." As you know by now, there isn't this one thing called "sex" you can consent to anyhow. "Sex" is an evolving series of actions and interactions. You have to have the enthusiastic consent of your partner for all of them. And even if you have your partner's consent for a particular activity, you have to be prepared for it to change.

"My partner and I were having sex in the missionary position, and I asked if we could switch to spooning," recalls Miranda, age nineteen. "He said yes, and we did. I was enjoying it quite a lot but couldn't get a read on him, so I asked, 'Does that feel good?' and he said, 'Yes, so good.' Such simple communication, but it really goes a long way towards ensuring mutual enjoyment."

Consent isn't a yes/no question. It's a state. If, instead of lovers, the two of you were synchronized swimmers, consent would be the water. It's not enough to jump in, get wet, and climb out—if you want to swim, you have to be in the water continually. And if you want to have sex, you have to be continually in a state of enthusiastic consent with your partner. That means you have to keep paying attention to your partner's verbal and nonverbal cues, and keep checking in if and when you can't tell.

Speaking of verbal and nonverbal cues, they can both count toward enthusiastic consent. As a general rule, I rely more heavily on verbal cues (you're looking for variations on the words "yes, please!" here) when I'm having sex with a new partner and trust myself more to correctly interpret nonverbal cues (like facial expressions, body language, and enthusiastic noises) when I'm with someone I've been intimate with for a while.

Of course, the real tricky part is this: However, well, *enthusiastic* you may be about practicing enthusiastic consent, your partners may not have ever heard of it or get why it's important. That can be challenging. You may need to discuss it with them and see what they think about it. But consider this question: Why would you want to have sex with someone who's not enthusiastic about it? Would you want to sleep with someone who doesn't care about whether or not you're into it?

Dive In: How do you define consent? Do you think you and your partners should just focus on stopping if someone says no, or do you think everyone should take responsibility for ensuring that their partner is actively enthusiastic about what's happening at all times? Write about consent in your notebook for ten minutes. Write about what you believe consent should involve, but also write about your experiences with saying yes and no to sex. When were you listened to? When weren't you?

HOT OR NOT

Telling your partner(s) what turns you on can feel terrifying if you haven't done it much before. It can feel incredibly vulnerable: *What if they laugh at me? What if they're disgusted? What if they turn me down?* Even before that, it requires you to admit aloud that you have desires—and not just generally "desire," which can be challenging enough, depending on your background, but specific, personal, sexual desires—ones that someone else should care about. Yeesh.

And yet. Like Mick Jagger sings in the old Stones classic, you can't always get what you want, but if you try sometimes, you just might find you get what you need. Or, as my mother always taught me about negotiations, "Ask. The worst they can do is say no."

Which is all to say, you picked up this book in order to find your way to a more fulfilling, you-centered sex life. And you can't get it if you don't tell your partner what you want in bed. You don't have to be bossy or insulting—offer suggestions in the spirit of collaboration, using the Nice Person Test. Don't you want to hear about things that would make your lover happy? Well, any good partner does, too. Don't assume that any of us feels like we know what we're doing, especially with a new lover.

Now, it's entirely possible that you want some things that make you nervous to talk about. Maybe you have fantasies or desires that seem taboo to you. We're going to get more into those in chapter 8, but for now, just know that you don't have to tell your partner everything at once. Start with stuff that seems less risky—that you like more pressure, or less, or a little over to the left? Yes, that's the spot. And if you were to go in kind of a circle? Ahhhhhh . . .

It's also likely that some of the time, you won't know what you like until you try it. Then the question becomes: Are you enthusiastic about finding out if you like it? If the answer is yes, let your partner know that while you're into trying it, you're not sure how you'll feel about whatever it is that you're doing. That way, your partner will be better prepared if you do wind up having a negative response. If you're not into even finding out if you like something, that may well be your intuition speaking. Don't let anyone talk you into trying things in bed if even the trying doesn't appeal.

Also, you can change your mind! Just because you ask your partner to go down on you doesn't mean you can't also say "stop." Maybe you thought you'd like it but it feels too intense. Maybe it felt great but now you want to do something different. Maybe you've got a leg cramp. Doesn't matter. Desires are always changeable and revocable. A good partner should understand that, but if you're not sure yours does, you can check in with them about that at any time.

"My partner and I both deal with chronic pain, and often when we are having sex, positions need to change often," says Jenn, age twenty-four.

> *At first, we were clumsy about it, and everything had to stop, and we'd reposition and have to get going again with diminished energy. When I'm the hurting party, I tend to just exclaim something ridiculous, like "ow" or "cramp!" and start laughing like crazy. We're at a point now where "ow" is not a problem word anymore, it's just a signal, and we laugh and keep going. What used to take what seemed like forever is now pretty seamless. The laughter helps.*

There's a flip side, too. Being comfortable with sexual communication is the only way to ensure you'll feel comfortable setting boundaries. If you can't talk about what you want, it makes it that much harder to talk about what you *don't* want. I know that I often hesitate a little bit before I set a sexual boundary, because I hate disappointing my partners. Thing is? They're hardly ever really disappointed, because I get sexual only with people who care whether or not I'm having a good time, and there are plenty of things we can do that make us both happy. But even if you're disappointing your partner, isn't that better than squelching your own desire and never trying to get it fulfilled?

Dive In: Fill out a Yes/No/Maybe list! The Yes/No/Maybe list was invented by the kinky community (more on that in chapter 8), but can be used by anyone. It's a list of sexual activities, and your job is to mark down one of three responses to each: Yes, I love (or would love) to do that; No, I really don't want to do that; or Maybe,

I'm not sure if I want to do that (or it depends on the circumstances). Y/N/M lists are a great way to get in touch with your turn-ons and turnoffs, the better to communicate them to your partner. So fill one out—this one is good for starters: www.wyrrw.com/ynm. (Note: All Y/N/M lists are likely to include sex acts that make you think, *Ew!* or, *Umm . . . people* do *that?* That's the point. Just say no to those. This isn't a dare, or a checklist of things you ought to want to do. It's just a way of getting to know your own desires better.)

Once you've done that, it's time for another practice conversation! Using any of the role-playing methods we went over earlier in the chapter, practice telling your partner (a real one or a hypothetical one) about one thing that turns you on and one thing that turns you off. If you're up to it, and you have a current sex partner or a friend who's willing, have them fill out the same Y/N/M list you did, and compare and discuss your answers.

SAFE IS SEXY

We talked about managing risk some in chapter 4, but now we're adding a new twist: another person to manage it with. Depending on your partner in play, that person can be an ally in keeping you both safe from STDs and pregnancy, or an obstacle. I encourage you to find out which one they are as soon as you can.

At risk of being redundant, I can tell you that it really does help to know what you want in terms of safer sex practices before you enter this negotiation. (For a comprehensive resource on your safer sex options, check out this Scarleteen article: www.wyrrw.com/safersex.)

Once you've got that down, the next step is to find out where your partner is at and what the two of you can agree on. You can do this up front, or you can do it as you go along (as your partner starts to go down on you, you could hand them a dental dam, for example).

Talking about STD status can be a little trickier. If you have an STD that your partner could catch, you have to decide if/when, and how to disclose that to your partner. We'll be diving into this in chapters 8 and 9, but I think the Golden Rule applies here: Do unto others as you'd have them do unto you. Wouldn't you rather know if you're at risk of catching something from having sex with your partner? Well, unless there are extenuating circumstances (like fear your safety will be at risk if you tell), that goes both ways.

One time I had a one-night stand where I brought someone home and things quickly got heated. Just as we were about to do something that involved swapping fluids—and as I was perched on top of them—they said, "When's the last time you were tested?" I had a pretty good idea of my status but had not ever been tested (fully because of my own fears), and my response was "I'm clean." We then proceeded to have a lot of unprotected sex. I consider myself extremely lucky that neither of us contracted anything from that experience, and frequently tell that story when I am speaking to youth about why it is so important to have safer sexual activity conversations prior to being in the heat of the moment. {Scout, twenty-five}

Even if you have no known diseases, it's a great idea to bring up the topic before you get naked, because you can't assume your partner will tell you if you don't ask. (It's also possible your partner will lie, which is yet another reason to practice safer sex even if neither of you has any known diseases, but most people will tell you what they know if asked directly.) It's hard to make questions about disease sexy, so it will feel more like an interruption of the mood the hotter and heavier you get. And there are some very particular questions to ask. Here's what I use:

- *Do you have any STDs?* If the answer is yes, ask follow-up questions about what your partner is doing about risk reduction, but also feel free to put off getting down until you do whatever research is necessary to make you feel comfortable with the risk. Or perhaps you'll decide you're not comfort- able with the risks, so sex is off the table with this person.

- *When was the last time you were tested?* Some STDs take up to six months to show up on tests and/or show symptoms. This means that even if the tests show your potential partner doesn't have HIV, they could have been exposed to it in the six-month period before they were tested, and it wouldn't show up on that test.

- *What have been your safer sex practices in the period the test doesn't cover?* Did you use those practices sometimes, or always? And do you know the STD status of whatever partners you've had in that period?

You're looking for two things when you ask these questions:

1. The actual information, which will help you decide how comfortable you are with the STD risks involved with sleeping with this particular person (remember that no partnered sex is zero risk).

2. The way they respond to the questions. Are they impatient with you, or direct and respectful? Someone who can't handle these questions is less likely to be handling their own STD prevention, either. But someone who is open and forthcoming (and asks you, too!) is likely to be someone you can trust to tell the truth and respect your safer sex needs.

As Prerna discovered, even decent partners can find this conversation challenging, but sticking with it can yield great results.

The first time I asked my boyfriend when he had been tested last, he was like, "Uh . . . never?" And I was like, "Well, you've had plenty of sexual partners, so you should probably do that." He was flustered by how direct I was, and by the fact that I was bringing it up at all. The next time, as I was going to visit him, I asked him if he'd gotten himself tested, and he said, "Well, I kinda forgot about it," and it was a really big internal struggle for me to then be like, Well, do I let that slide? But this is something that's really important to me. He's probably fine, but what if he's not? I don't know his former partners. So I stuck to my guns about that. And he did get tested.

> **Dive In:** You guessed it: Practice having this conversation using your chosen role-playing method. Do it a few times, asking your conversation partner to give different kinds of answers each time—the kind of answers you hope to hear, the kind you fear you'll hear, perhaps answers you've received before but wish you'd responded differently to. Do it until you feel comfortable saying what you need to to feel safe and in control in the situation.

DIRTY TALK

All of this talking-about-sex stuff is hard, in part because most of us have been trained not to talk about sex, and especially not to talk about it with our sexual partners, and *absolutely* not to talk about it with our partners while we're actually *having* sex. This is profoundly damaging, yes, but also profoundly silly. Sex talk can be hot! There's a whole industry devoted to providing people with the opportunity to get off while talking about sex, an industry that nets phone companies an estimated $500 million annually.[2] Sex talk is obviously appealing to a whole lot of people.

Direct talk about sex has the unearned reputation of being antisexy, but the truth is that much of the communication I'm suggesting in this chapter can be done in a way that makes you and your partner hotter for each other. And I don't just mean talking about what turns you on, though seriously, that can be a sexy-as-hell conversation, too. Want to check if you've got enthusiastic consent? Try asking in a sexy voice: "Do you like it when I do that? Does that feel good? I really want to do X; do you want me to?" You get the idea—it doesn't have to sound like you're negotiating a contract. The important thing is to be clear and make sure you get an answer. And ask again when you're moving on to a new sex act.

Even boundary setting doesn't have to kill a mood. If you want your partner to stop doing a particular thing but you still want the general sexytime to continue, try suggesting a hot alternative. Instead of just saying, "Can you stop? I don't like that," try, "Could we do this other awesome thing now?" Use a commanding voice, or a begging voice, or whatever voice makes you feel sexy.

And if you try to say something sexy and it comes out sounding silly and you both giggle? Have fun with it. Sex can be silly, too. Enjoy the laugh, and then double down by saying something even dirtier.

The first time I hooked up with my ex, we were at a small party. We started cuddling, and then the chemistry just hit us. He was wearing a shirt that said MENOTOMY ROCKS—Menotomy is the name of a local park—so I started joking that his Menotomy was showing, which led to all sorts of geographical innuendoes. At one point, I was even making sexual references to the Boston subway lines—"getting off at Longwood," "riding the blue line all the way to Wonderland," etc. It was so wonderful and silly and unexpectedly hot! {Laura, twenty-five}

> **Dive In:** Get down 'n' dirty with your last practice conversation of the week. Make a list of the kinds of sexual conversations that make you nervous, then pick one and practice doing it sexy-style. Have fun with it. There are lots of ways to sound sexy. Try on approaches you've seen in movies or books; get advice from your friends if you feel comfortable. Try approaches that seem totally opposite from what you usually do. Be playful with this exercise. Don't be afraid to laugh. But don't be afraid to get serious, either.

IF IT DOESN'T GO WELL

Of course, there is always the potential that you'll do your very best job communicating something you want or need and your partner won't respond well. Sometimes your partner may see your comments or requests as criticism of their performance, rather than expressions of how and where you prefer to be touched, kissed, or penetrated. Some people have the unreasonable expectation that they shouldn't have to be told what to do, and if they do, it's a challenge to their sexual prowess. Others may simply take it too personally and have their feelings hurt. Thus, your lover may get defensive, or burst into tears, or make fun of you, or try to pressure you to change your mind, or ignore you altogether.

I can't tell you how to make that not feel bad for *you*, too: You're putting yourself out there, and you're getting blowback in return. But I can tell you that it probably has nothing at all to do with you. If you're being direct and respectful, and you get static as a result, that tells you volumes more about your partner than it does about you.

Joey, twenty-six, has struggled with this firsthand.

My first sexual partner had an aversion to condoms. I have a history of sexual abuse, so it was hard for me in the beginning to be assertive and make myself heard. I tried several times to start a conversation with him about safer sex, but he always managed to make me feel like I was somehow being a prude or a worrywart. In the end, I bought a box of condoms and told him it was either that or no sex. Needless to say, the relationship didn't last long.

Your partner's response can be hard to take. None of us want to suddenly realize we're with a partner whom we can't trust to be caring with us when we're being open or even vulnerable with them. It can take a lot of courage to put yourself out there like this, and negative responses can be mortifying and discouraging. At worst it can be a heartbreaking loss, seeming to confirm our fears that no one good will ever want or love us.

That's why the first thing to do if it doesn't go well is to consider the circumstances. Is this kind of behavior a pattern, or is this an isolated incident? Could my partner be having a bad day, or responding to something that has nothing to do with me? Don't make excuses—try to answer these questions for yourself as honestly as possible. But don't jump to the worst conclusion, either. (Incidentally, these questions are clearly easier to answer the better you know your partner, which is one of the factors that can make sex with someone you don't know much more challenging to navigate than sex with someone you're closer to.)

But if you suspect this response doesn't stem from extenuating circumstances, do your best to consider it a gift—the gift of information. If your partner can't handle direct, respectful sexual communication, it may mean they're not a very safe person to be intimate with. I'm not just talking about whether they ignore your physical boundaries. If your partner mocks or dismisses your desires, or pressures you to forgo safe sex, or ignores your concerns about STDs, or is uninterested in your emotional state, that's a partner who's not interested in helping you get what you really really want. It may be a partner who's going to actively prevent you from getting it, keeping you off-center and unfulfilled as a way of controlling you. It may be a partner who is going to be callous and cold and hurt you without even caring. It may be a partner who's too insecure and needy to respect you as a person, instead focusing only on what you can give to them.

Whatever the case, please believe me when I say you deserve better. (You may still be in the process of coming to believe that yourself. If you feel shaky about that idea, go revisit all the work you just did in chapters 4, 5, and 6.) You deserve a partner who is going to help you get what you really really want. And if you give your energy to people who are ignoring or working against that goal, not only are you teaching yourself that their behavior is okay, but you're also so busy dealing with people who aren't treating you right that you're missing opportunities to meet someone better.

Dive In: Get out your timeline, and add some times when you tried to tell a partner something important about sex and it didn't go well. Then add a few times when you did the same thing and it was well received. Pick one example of each, and write about them. What did each incident have in common, and what was different? Did your communication style make a difference, or the subject matter? In retrospect, what do you think your partners' responses reveal about them and about your relationship?

BE KIND TO YOURSELF

Don't forget that this is *not* a test. The point of all of this communication is to decrease your risk of emotional or physical harm and increase your pleasure! Do your best, and you'll improve over time, but you'll never be perfect. You'll get carried away in the heat of the moment and forget to ask about your partner's STD status or their expectations. You'll desperately want to ask a partner to do something you really really want, but you'll get shy and stay mum. You'll squelch your need to set a boundary because you're afraid of how your partner will respond. Don't worry. I still do all of these things on occasion, and you will, too. Be kind to yourself.

It probably won't be the end of the world, but if there are consequences for not communicating (for example, you get pregnant accidentally, or you feel gross because you let your partner think you were into something when you weren't), deal with it as directly and lovingly as you can. Blaming yourself will not heal you faster. If there are consequences to your part-ner (you give them an STD, you find out that they felt violated because you didn't ensure they were enthusiastically consent-ing), that's a little more complicated. We'll be talking about that in chapter 9.

Most of the time, if your intentions are good but you act on them imperfectly, it will be all right. Just notice that it hap-pened, check in with yourself about it, and think about how/ if you'd like to handle things differently the next time. Then let it go. The point of all this is to do your best on your own behalf and on behalf of your partner. That's all we can ask of ourselves.

Go Deeper:

1. **Write a graphic sex scene.** A lot of literary sex scenes are kind of vague and woolly. Others sound like medical dictionaries. Write a killer sex scene that is really specific. Start with what would turn you on in terms of flirting—a great meal (but what is a great meal for you?), a conversation (about what?), a hot night on the dance floor (what song is playing? What are you both wear-ing?), a hike or a walk with the dogs (how do your dogs get along?).

   Who makes the first move, and how? What do you talk about, if anything? How does your lover react, respond, or behave? How do you each know that you are consenting enthusiastically? Try to show the signals, verbal or nonverbal, that might be exchanged in the awesome dance of sex.

Take it from there. Fulfill some long-held fantasies. Write a great sex scene. Then: What do you do, or say, afterward?

2. Write about bad sex. Write about a mercy fuck, or a bad mistake, or breakup sex, or angry sex, or even indifferent sex. It can be funny. It can also be tragic or painful. As with the above, go into detail. What was so bad, or so funny? Did your belts get tangled? Did the dogs watch? Did your mother call in the middle of the action?

   Call it like you see it. You don't need to show it to anyone, ever.

3. Rewrite the script. Have you had bad experiences trying to communicate your desires and limits to a partner? You can't make someone respond the way you want them to in real life, but you can in this exercise. Pick one of the times you identified in the timeline exercise earlier in the chapter, and use your dominant hand to write the parts you said or wish you'd said, and then use your non-dominant hand to respond the way you would ideally like a partner to respond. Or, if you'd rather, use any of the role-playing techniques from this chapter to play out a different ending, and just make sure to tell your role-play partner how you want them to respond!

CHAPTER 8

IT'S COMPLICATED

N OW THAT YOU'RE LEARNING TO MASTER THE BASICS OF sexual communication, it's time to talk about sex itself—or rather, common sexual situations that can, well, make things a little more complicated. As you'll find, as long as you have access to accurate information; stay in touch with your needs, desires, and boundaries; remember your risk assessment tools; and use direct communication, you'll be able to manage whatever challenges come your way on the road to what you really really want.

But before we get messy, check in: How are you doing with your daily writing? Are you still practicing weekly body love? The more complicated that things get, the more important it is to use these simple rituals to stay grounded.

ARE THERE RULES?

When it comes to pursuing and enjoying sexual relationships, nearly everyone will tell you that you've got to play a good game. Trouble is, no one can agree on the rules. Don't call him; let him call you. Never have sex before the third date. Laugh at all her jokes, even if you don't really think they're funny. There are so many rules that you never ever know if your rules match the rules of the person you're trying to play "the game" with. It's entirely possible that you don't even agree on what the prize is if you win. Which is why you should play only by rules that make sense to *you*, whether or not your prospective partner agrees.

In other words: Don't play games because you think you have to, or you're expected to, or no one will want you otherwise. It's bunk. In all likelihood, the object of your affection is trying to figure out what rules you're playing by so they can play by them, too, causing the two of you to circle each other in an endless loop of second-guessing. What's worse, even if you do manage to attract someone's attention by playing what you've convinced yourself is the right game, you won't know if that person is actually attracted to you, because you won't be acting from an authentic place.

(It's worth also saying that you shouldn't play games in order to manipulate or control your partner, either. We'll be talking more about that in chapter 9.)

You want to play flirty, coy games because they're fun for you? Have at it. You want to be a bold seductress or play hard to get because that dynamic turns you on? Go for it. But make sure you're acting on behalf of yourself, in pursuit of what you really really want. In all things, be real. Even if you're playing games.

Dive In: Make a list of sexual rules that make sense to you. They can be specific and directive ("No oral sex for people who won't reciprocate"), general guidelines ("Whatever I do is okay, as long as I feel safe"), or more creative ("When all else fails, I ask myself: What Would Cleopatra Do?"). Have fun!

THE BLOWJOB PARADOX

Riddle me this: Why are women who give blowjobs often treated as though they're doing something demeaning, while men receiving those blowjobs are seen as doing something awesome? For that matter, why do we have the same attitude toward women who are on the receiving end of anal sex, or who "tea bag" (put a guy's balls in their mouth)? And why are those same activities—receiving anal sex and performing oral sex (especially on other men) considered "feminine" and demeaning when men do them? This, my friends, is the "blowjob paradox."

Time and again, our culture treats the traditionally "female" role as one to avoid. You can even see it in our curse words: Why is being a cocksucker a bad thing? Why is someone who's been taken advantage of said to have been "fucked over"? And someone who's had a bad situation forced on them told they've had to "take it up the ass"? What about when guys bully other guys for being weak or timid by calling them "pussies"? And, by the same token, say someone has "balls" if they're assertive and strong? It all stems from the idea that women should neither enthusiastically enjoy sex nor be assertive about our desire, so if we've agreed to do anything more creative than "lie back and think of England," we've obviously been forced to do it in order to please a man.

There's nothing inherently demeaning about a blowjob (or any other sexual activity, for that matter). As long as both partners are enthusiastically consenting, why would one person be degraded and the other elevated? Besides, blowjobs aren't even necessarily submissive—it's all in how you and your partner approach them. As Gray puts it, "In my mind, if I'm doing something to someone that's making their toes curl, I consider myself the person in power. I am the person doing things. I'm the active agent."

Blowjobs (and other "coded female" sex acts) are only demeaning if you or your partner experiences them as such. If you feel like you have no choice but to give your partner a blowjob, even though you don't want to? That's degrading. But it has nothing to do with cocksucking itself, and everything to do with the way your partner is treating you.

> **Dive In:** Make a list of sex acts that you've seen treated as demeaning or degrading. Now pick one you enjoy, or think you would enjoy. Spend five minutes writing about that sex act. What do you like about it? How does (or would) it make you feel? Don't hold back: Be as elaborately specific as you can, and as enthusiastic as you want to be. When you feel you've run out of things to say, complete this sentence: There's one more thing I want to say about this, and it's:_____.

BAD KISSING (AND OTHER MISFORTUNES)

So. You're on a date, or hanging out with the object of your affection. Maybe it's been an hour, maybe it's been a week, maybe it's been a year, but for however long, you've known. You've just known you want to kiss this person. And then the moment finally arrives, and you lean in, and the music in your mind swells, and your lips touch and . . .

Ick. Too slobbery, too dry, funny tasting, bad breath, too tense, too aggressive, too flaccid—whatever the problem, a bad kiss is like an off-season tomato—it can be worse than no kiss at all.

The really tricky thing about a bad kiss is what happens next. Since you've gotten this far in the book, it probably won't surprise you at this point that the answer is "it depends." More specifically, it depends on three things:

1. How invested are you in this person?

The more invested you are in developing a sexual or romantic relationship with the Bad Kisser, the more motivated you'll be to somehow get past the bad kissing.

2. How likely are you to be able to improve the situation?

Age and experience are two factors when it comes to an individual's willingness to improve their smoochability. But you also have to consider their personality and temperament. Are they curious by nature? Do they like to try new things? How much of their ego is invested in being "good" at sexual or romantic things? Also, consider your relationship. Do you already trust each other? Are you someone from whom this person can take careful criticism?

3. How bad is the kissing, really?

Is it just a slightly disappointing kiss, perhaps paling in comparison with one from a champion kisser you've locked lips with before? Or is it a big problem, the kind that makes your body tense up and all your circuits sound the alarm?

Whatever your answers are to those three questions, you've got three options for action:

1. Suck it up.

Maybe you're madly in love with this person already and the problem isn't all that bad. Or maybe it *is* that bad but your desire to be with them trumps whatever the problem is. Sometimes the person of your dreams may have a subpar pucker. There are worse things that could happen.

2. Try to change it.

So, you don't want to bail on the person, but the problem is bad enough that you don't want to live with it, either. Like any criticism, it will go down better with a spoonful of sugar. I like to use the "shit sandwich" method, which involves wedging whatever challenging feedback you need to convey between two slices of positive affirmation. In this case, that might sound something like this: "I really love being close to you. But I've noticed, when we kiss? You kind of tense up your lips. Do you think you could try to relax them more, so that I can really feel how soft and delicious they are?"

See what I did there? Nothing makes difficult news go down more easily than compliments. Just make sure to pick some that you mean—nothing makes difficult news go down worse than false sentiment.

Another thing to note about what I did in that example is that I got very specific. I didn't say, "You kiss kinda funny." I didn't even say, "Can you just chill out more?" I was very specific both about what was going wrong for me and about how I hoped it could go differently. This gives your partner something concrete to work with, and it also helps them avoid feeling like they're just terrible at kissing in general.

A lot of mistakes people make in the kissing department may be related to performance anxiety. Ideally, sexual interactions should be more like playful explorations and improvisational communication than like some kind of judged Olympic competition, but the reality is that your partner may have absorbed messages to the contrary.

Which is a great point to keep in mind if your partner takes your feedback badly. If this happens, reassure your partner that kissing preferences are totally subjective! You're not saying they are *bad* at kissing, you're just saying that you would like kissing even better if they considered trying it a new way.

If that doesn't work, you may have to backpedal, or you might have to sit down and really hash things out. Be empathetic—nobody wants to hear they don't make you weak in the knees—but don't forget that it's important to speak up for your needs in a sexual relationship, as long as you do so in a spirit of respect and collaboration. If you approach it that way, and if your partner takes the same approach, this is a mere bump in the road, even if it feels a little rocky at the time. And if your partner can't deal with the fact that they aren't utterly perfect, perhaps they're not the best partner for you after all.

3. That brings us to your third option: Leave.

If you're not that invested in this partner, or if kissing is really that bad, it's totally legitimate to move on. Chemistry is important. If you kiss someone and it doesn't make you want to kiss them more? Maybe you shouldn't be kissing that person. It doesn't mean they're not a good person, or that you don't find them attractive. It simply means something's not aligned sexually between you.

Pushing yourself to be attracted to someone can lead to a situation where you're in an emotionally committed relationship but your desire has died out or dwindled. And that's a much harder problem to deal with than coming to terms with the fact that a person you thought you might have a spark with isn't making you spark enough.

Of course, if you're calling something off because the kissing isn't right, the kind thing to do is not to say this explicitly. Try saying something more general but still true—again, using a shit sandwich. For example: "I just wanted to say that I've been having a great time getting to know you, but I'm just not feeling the chemistry I'm looking for. I'm disappointed, actually, because you're such an excellent person otherwise." At which point you could even share a couple examples of things you like about the person.

You've probably realized that all of this kissing-compatibility advice isn't limited just to kissing. Sexual desire is a complex and personal thing. Much like a fingerprint, it's hard to imagine two people wanting the exact same things the exact same ways at all times, sexually speaking. Negotiating the difference between what you want and what your partner wants is a healthy and crucial thing to do. The key is being able to communicate about it. And the kissing principles are good ones to guide you, whatever the issue.

Dive In: Get out your timeline and add some sexual situations you've been in where the compatibility just wasn't where you wanted it to be. Now pick one that you still have feelings about, and write about it in your journal: How did you handle it? How did the other person handle it? How did your approach work or not work? Would you do anything differently if you had it to do over? If so, write an alternate story in which you do it the way you wish you could have. Write it as though it really happened that way. How does that change things?

WHEN YOU AND YOUR BODY DISAGREE

This is a tough one, largely because it's hard to talk about our bodies' being separate from ourselves. Because they're not really, are they? Anything that happens to our bodies happens to us, and it's a scientific fact that how we're feeling emotionally can affect our physical health. We're pretty connected to our bodies, and yet sometimes our bodies can feel pretty alien. And that's confusing, to say the least.

The most extreme example of this is how some people's bodies respond to sexual violence. Both men and women can, if being sexually assaulted, show signs of arousal. In most women, that means that your vagina may lubricate, your nipples may harden—some people even have an orgasm.

Does their physical response mean they're consenting to sex? Of course not. There are many theories about why this happens, a popular one being that the body is protecting itself, as a lubricated vagina is less likely to tear or otherwise be physically hurt when something is inserted into it. Whatever the reason, your body may feel turned on when the rest of you doesn't. That doesn't mean you're consenting to anything, much less enthusiastic about it. Real enthusiastic consent happens only when your body and mind are in agreement.

This body-self disconnect can happen in reverse, too. Have you ever liked—even adored—someone so much but weren't attracted to them, despite how much you wished you would be? Or do you ever find yourself physically attracted to someone you would never want to trust with your emotional safety? That's your body being out of sync in a different way. There's nothing wrong with you if this happens, but it is important to avoid trying to convince yourself that you're attracted to someone just because you think they're terrific otherwise, or because you'd like to avoid hurting their feelings by rejecting them.

Sometimes your body will just go one way when the rest of you goes another. That can be kind of confusing, but it's perfectly normal. Because while your body is a part of who you are, it's not all of you. You get to decide what to do if this split occurs: have a hot fling with someone you want no ongoing emotional relationship with? Invest in a friendship and hope attraction follows? Walk on by, because you want all or nothing? They're all valid decisions.

On the other hand, if you find that you regularly part ways with your body—say, you hardly ever find yourself physically attracted to someone you actually like as a person, and vice versa—that may be a sign that something larger is amiss, especially if it bothers you. It might signify an attraction to people who treat you badly, which can be a sign that, deep down, that's how you believe you should be treated, or that's how you're used to being treated, so it feels comfortable. It can also be a sign that you're afraid of being close to someone in a romantic relationship—that physical intimacy combined with emotional intimacy is too intense for you. If that's the case, you may have some generalized fears to work through from previous emotional injuries. Therapy or counseling can be very useful for addressing these issues, if you have access to it.

> **Dive In:** Write down a few times when your body and the rest of you went different ways. Then pick one and write about it a little, with your dominant hand writing for your body and your nondominant hand writing for the rest of you. Let each of them explain what they wanted in the situation, and why. Let them argue with each other if they want to. Then see if they can come to an agreement about anything related to the situation.

KINKS/BDSM

You've probably heard the word "kinky" before. You may or may not know the term "BDSM." Depending on whom you ask, it stands for some variation of the terms "bondage," "discipline," "domination," "submission," "sadism," and "masochism."

If you feel confused or ashamed because you get turned on by things (or even just the fantasies of things) that you "shouldn't" be turned on by, the first thing I can tell you is that you're far from alone. You'd be surprised how many people have "nontraditional" desires. These include wanting to do any of the following: have power over someone, surrender power, be tied up (bondage) or do the tying, have sex in public places (like a dressing room or a train), receive or administer pain (consensually, of course!), verbally degrade your partner or be degraded . . . the list goes on, and this is just the tip of the iceberg. If you feel like a freak because you want something "weird," you are not alone. There are many people out there who want the same thing.

One of the most challenging parts of being kinky is that our desires may not match up with our ideals. For example, like most women, you believe that we should be treated with respect by our lovers. And yet you may also, in the privacy of your sexual space, want your lover to do some things that may seem very disrespectful. Like call you a dirty little slut, for example. Or tie you to the bed. Or spank you. Or maybe you want to do these things to others.

Renee, thirty-one, encountered this tension when she met a man who liked to take the reins:

I found his dominance to be quite a turn-on. This con-fused me a great deal, because I am a strong feminist and exercise power in my daily life better than just about anybody I know. Yet this opportunity to relinquish control intrigued me, and soon this man and I began writing out fantasies to each other in which he dominated me. It was the writing itself that helped me come to terms with this fantasy, sometimes involving ropes, blindfolds, or, in one he wrote, even scissors. What I eventually realized is that creating scenarios in which I surrender my power can be among my most powerful acts. I also figured out a line in my head, which is that while power turns me on, abuse of power does not. In order to surrender in this way, I must be met with love.

The conflict between philosophy and desire can feel charged—and perhaps more so if you're a survivor of sexual violence and your fantasies run violent. If this tension is troubling you, it may be time for a reframe. Try thinking of sex as a playspace for adults. Time to explore worlds that aren't real, and perhaps help us process the world around us. Remember when you were a kid on the playground and you'd create entire imaginary worlds and assign each other roles to play? When I was growing up, sometimes we'd take on roles from TV and movies, or make up wild imaginary worlds, or act out variations on themes from the real world, like playing "house" or "office." Ultimately, we were stepping out of our own reality to see the world from a different perspective—to simultaneously expand and escape our world by breaking its rules.

Sex can be like that, and kinky sex especially—a place to experiment with power, sensation, characters, and experiences that aren't possible in the rest of your life. Maybe you find it hard to relinquish control most of the time, and sex play affords you the chance to experience helplessness. Or the opposite could be true—it could give you the chance to finally be as in control of everything as you always wished you could be.

Additionally, some survivors of violence find it cathartic to play out "scenes" similar to how they were violated, but in a safe space, with someone they trust, and with the option of calling a stop to the action at any time. That option is not a negligible detail here—psychologically, exploring an old dynamic safely and with new power can be pretty healing. Even if you've never been sexually violated, your sex life can be a safe space to explore what can be dangerous or terrifying in real life.

Of course, the key word in that last sentence is "safe." When you're playing with power and/or pain, it's crucial to be able to tell whom you can trust. Responsible kinksters—just like all responsible lovers—are the ones who are interested in your desires, patient with your questions, invested in your safety, and respectful of your boundaries. These folks often rely on a simple motto to guide them: All of their activities should be "safe, sane, and consensual." By now, you're probably on your way to developing your own definitions of these words, and tools with which to ensure you and your partners are abiding by them, which is great. To those definitions and tools I'll add one more that's kink-specific: the safeword.

The basic idea of a safeword is this: It's a word you or your partner can use to withdraw consent if you've negotiated a scene in which "no" no longer means no. (People sometimes do this in order to play with the dynamics of helplessness and control.) If you're playing this way, it's important to have another word—a word unlikely to come up accidentally—that will let the partner in control know that the partner who's submitting wants to stop. You can use a random, easy-to-remember word that you agree on in advance (like "tofu" or "bubbles" or whatever you like), or you can use the green/yellow/red model, where if you're fully enthusiastic about what's happening and your partner checks in, you say "green"; if you're starting to reach your limit but don't want the action to stop yet, you can let your partner know by saying "yellow"; and if you want to stop you say "red."

And safewords are just the tip of the iceberg when it comes to what kinksters have developed to help encourage folks to engage in direct sexual communication. Says Heidi,

> As I've gotten more involved in the S&M scene, I've realized that there's no real room for hiding your voice in this community. Because it's like, no, you need to figure out what you want and how far you want to go. You have to negotiate terms beforehand, which isn't something I'm used to. I tend to be like, "Oh, whatever you want." And that just doesn't work here. It's really helping me improve communication with potential partners.

In other words: Whether or not your own desires run kinky, there are many ways we can learn from the BDSM community about how best to get what we really really want.

> **Dive In:** There's a big difference between knowing hypothetically that lots of people are kinky in one way or another and actually connecting with people who practice in a healthy way. Even if you're not kinky yourself, there's a lot you can learn from folks who know how to explicitly negotiate pleasure and safety. This week, get more familiar with what's out there and who's doing it. Spend at least thirty minutes exploring one or more of the following resources:
>
> - A Kink 101 collection: www.wyrrw.com/kink101
> - Clarisse Thorn's Greatest Hits: www.wyrrw.com/clarissethorn
> - Carnival of Kinky Feminists: www.wyrrw.com/kinkcarnival
> - *Screw the Roses, Send Me the Thorns,* by Philip Miller and Molly Devon
> - *The New Topping Book* and/or *The New Bottoming Book,* both by Janet Hardy and Dossie Easton
> - FetLife.com[1]

FANTASY VS. REALITY

Of course, sometimes a fantasy is just that: a flight of the imagination. It can be hard to tell which of your fantasies you want to make real and which are better left as masturbation fodder.

There's no great way to tell without trying. But you don't have to jump in with both feet, either. If you want to explore bringing a fantasy into your sex life, try talking about it with your partner while you're being sexual. See how you feel—does imagining it together make the experience hotter, or does it make you freeze up or back off? If it gets your blood flowing, try a next, interim step. For example, if you fantasize about tying someone up, see how it feels just to hold them down or loop a scarf loosely around their wrists—something you can back away from quickly if it winds up feeling bad. (Ensure your partner's enthusiastic consent before trying this, of course!) If it feels good and you're both still into it, you can go on upping the ante until you're playing out your fantasy, or until you or a partner hits a comfort threshold.

Rachel, age twenty, learned about diving in too fast when she tried out a fantasy of hers: sex while high. "I had heard it increased sensation and was generally fun, so I brought it up with my girlfriend," she remembers.

It was something she had also wanted to try. We ate pot brownies, cuddled, and got to business. I had apparently eaten way too much of the brownie, because I periodically forgot who my girlfriend was and what was happening. I kept thinking she might be the man who sexually assaulted me. We stopped, and luckily I didn't have a full-blown panic attack, but it's not something I've ever wanted to try again.

It's also important to consider *whose* fantasies you're bringing to life. This question goes all the way back to chapters 1 and 3, in which you considered the many influences that have shaped how you think about sexuality and started to adjust them so that they sounded more like you and less like other people's agendas for you. Hopefully you've got that balance much closer to where you want it to be by now, but when it comes to fantasy, it's good to check in. Because the virgin/slut dichotomy is so ingrained in our culture, women with whom the "innocent" label doesn't resonate may believe that the only other valid option for expressing their sexuality is to be as "wild," sexually speaking, as possible. As I've said before, there's nothing wrong with being sexually wild, as long as you're doing it on your own terms and taking on only the risks you're comfortable with. You don't have to be "up for anything" in order to be loved, or to find a satisfying sex partner. Your satisfaction depends on your developing a specific, authentic sexual identity and finding partners that want you where you are, as opposed to expecting you to fit some kind of porn-fueled fantasy of what a sexual woman should be like. Yet another reason to take it one step at a time when exploring fantasies—you may find out along the way that they don't belong to you in the first place.

You may also find that some fantasies feel great when you're enacting them, but not so good afterward. It's hard to know when or why this will happen. For some, playing with fantasy dynamics that would be toxic if they were "real" can be liberating and satisfying, and for others, these same play dynamics (say, having your lover say humiliating things to you) may feel hot at the time but can wind up reinforcing the damaging beliefs you have about yourself that you're trying to shed. If you find this to be true, it's important to include that in your risk assessment when considering whether and how to play with that dynamic again.

Dive In: Write a list of five sexual fantasies that you've never tried in reality. Circle the one that turns you on the most when you think about it and the one that scares you the most. (They may be the same one, or different ones.) Now pick one of the ones you've circled, and write out a plan for trying it with a partner. What would your first step be? If that feels good, what would be the second step? How would you know if you and your partner each wanted to try more, and how would you know when you'd had enough? What are the risks in trying out your fantasy, and how can they be managed or minimized? What are the potential rewards?

DISCLOSING

Do you ever struggle with sharing information with your partner in terms of your sex life? Maybe it's admitting to a fantasy. Or telling them you have an STD. Maybe it's disclosing a trauma history, or your insecurity about being less experienced than your partner expects, or *more* experienced. Perhaps you're a sex worker, or used to be one. Maybe you're transgender. Maybe you have a mental or physical situation that's not readily apparent but will affect the way you have sex. Maybe it's something else entirely.

If this is the case, and you worry that your partner will respond poorly to your disclosure, these questions can be useful and clarifying:

- What are the risks to me if I bring this up? How likely are those risks to happen? Are there ways to reduce those risks?

- What are the risks to me if I don't bring this up before we have sex? How likely are those risks to happen? Are there ways to reduce those risks without telling my partner about this?

- What are the risks to my partner if I don't bring this up before we have sex? How likely are those risks to happen? Are there ways to reduce those risks without telling my partner about this?

- What are the benefits to me if I bring this up before we have sex? What about during? What about after or later? What are the benefits to me if I never bring it up?

Sound familiar? You're basically doing a risk analysis, just as you would for any other risky situation. And don't forget what you already know about risk: Every sexual scenario carries some. The question is, which risks seem like the right ones for you? And how can you minimize them?

In a practical sense, I encourage you to be honest with your partner when it seems possible. Lying is usually wrong, and hiding things can be exhausting. Disclosure gives you the opportunity to learn things about your partner. Do you want to be with someone who responds badly when you've shared something personal and important? On the other hand, if your partner responds well, it can build trust and intimacy between you, which can make sex better and strengthen your connection—whether it's a long-term affair or a fleeting hookup.

How and when to disclose depends on how urgent and risky the matter is. Unfortunately, those two often go hand in hand. One thing I've had to disclose for a long time is that I'm a survivor of sexual assault. At first, when I was just starting to have sex again after the assault, it was extremely important to me to tell partners about it before we did anything sexual. I felt fragile and volatile; I wanted to start reclaiming my body and sexuality, but I never knew when some small moment or gesture would trigger trauma memories. But at the same time, it was terrifying to tell partners so soon, because how they reacted mattered a lot to me. Today, eighteen years later, it's both less risky and less urgent for me to share.

Dive In: Write a list of any things about you that you'd prefer your sex partners to know but that are sometimes challenging for you to disclose. Then do a risk assessment on each of them, using the questions above. Be as detailed as you can be. Once you've completed that, write out what you think is the best time and approach to disclose to your partners. Then write a backup plan: If you don't achieve your ideal, for any reason, what's the next-best approach?

UNWANTED PAIN

For some of us, the obstacles to satisfying sex are more physical. Some people experience mild to intense pain when anything is inserted into their vagina. If you've tried vaginal penetration more than once and it just consistently hurts, you may be suffering from one of several very real medical conditions, including vulvodynia or vaginismus. If you suspect this might be the case for you, the first thing you should remember is that vaginal penetration isn't the only way to have sex! Experiment with other ways to please yourself and your lover. In the meantime, seek out medical help, because there are treatments available that can reduce or eliminate your pain. You may have to be persistent—not all doctors are familiar with these conditions or know how to treat them. For a listing of doctors that women have found helpful, as well as other resources, information, and support, I encourage you to check out www.wyrrw .com/vulvodynia or the book *Healing Sexual Pain,* by Deborah Coady, MD, and Nancy Fish, MPH.

The other common cause of unwanted physical pain during sex is anal sex. If you're the "enveloping" or "receiving" partner during anal sex and it hurts, one of several things may be amiss:

1. *You're not using enough lube.* There's no such thing as too much lube when it comes to anal sex! But be sure to use a water- or silicone-based lube if you're using a condom—oil-based lube will break down the latex and make it useless as a safer-sex barrier.

2. *You may not be relaxed enough, and/or you may be going too fast.* If you're enthusiastic about trying

anal sex but you find that it hurts, you may need to take it a little slower. Start with one finger, just in the anal opening. Go slowly and gradually, and make sure the penetrating partner backs off any time there's pain. (If your partner won't do that, they may not be a good partner to have anal sex with.) Take your time.

3. *You may be under pressure.* Check in with yourself: Is this something you really want for yourself? Or is this solely your partner's agenda? A good partner won't push you into doing anything you don't want to do and certainly won't encourage you to keep doing anything that causes unwanted pain.

4. *You may have a hemorrhoid (a swollen vein in the anal area) or a tear in the anal lining.* If you suspect this is the case—especially if there's blood—go see your doctor. These are very treatable conditions, as long as you don't exacerbate them with the friction of anal sex.

If you want to learn more about how to have pleasurable and painless anal sex, check out Tristan Taormino's *The Ultimate Guide to Anal Sex for Women.*

Dive In: If you're experiencing unwanted pain during sex—even a kind of pain not described here—please use the resources above to get help (including Scarleteen's Find-a-Doc service: www.wyrrw.com/scarleteenfindadoc), and keep trying new things until the pain stops. Everyone deserves a sex life free of unwanted pain.

IF YOU'VE BEEN VIOLATED

If someone violates your sexual boundaries, it can feel unspeakably awful. It can also be incredibly confusing if it's someone you trusted enough to have been voluntarily intimate with them. There are entire books about how to recover from sexual violence, including Ellen Bass's *The Courage to Heal* and Staci Haines's *Healing Sex,* but I want to mention a few things here:

It's not your fault. Not if you were wearing something sexy, or were drunk, or were walking alone by yourself at night. Not if you were flirting with someone, or making out with them, or naked, or fooling around. Nothing you do can ever make sexual violence your fault. If someone ignores your protests, or even doesn't care enough to notice that you've stopped enjoying or participating in whatever is happening, it's their fault. Always.

Tell someone. Seriously. Long before you were assaulted, you were taught that girls and women who get assaulted should feel shame. And that shame may discourage you from telling anyone what happened. But you have done nothing to be ashamed of. The person who violated your body should be ashamed, not you. Don't let that misplaced shame keep you from getting the support you need or the justice you deserve.

If you're sexually assaulted by someone you know or your attacker doesn't fit the stereotype of a "real" rapist—a brutal, violent stranger who tackles you from behind—you may also feel that it somehow "doesn't count" or isn't important enough to warrant anyone's concern. Many survivors of sexual violence do this to themselves, in part due to myths about how rape really happens (as we discussed in chapter 3, most of the time it's perpetrated by someone you know, not the stranger jumping out of the bushes we've been taught to fear), and in part as a way to keep us from holding perpetrators accountable. But every sexual violation is one too many, and every survivor is important. So please: *Tell* someone. Silence doesn't negate that it happened. Keeping quiet won't make you suffer any less, but it may make you suffer more, because you'll be suffering alone. I have heard so many heartbreaking stories of women who don't tell anyone for years, and their accrued pain is overwhelming.

Pick someone you think is likely to give you the support and unconditional acceptance that you need. If you don't know whom to call, a good place to start is RAINN (the Rape, Abuse & Incest National Network), which runs a U.S. phone hotline at (800) 656-HOPE and an access-from-anywhere web hotline at www.rainn.org.

You deserve justice. Depending on where you live and what was done to you, you have legal rights to file criminal charges and to sue for compensation for your pain and suffering. Learning more about your legal options doesn't lock you into action; it just gives you more choice and more control in the aftermath of an experience that may well have left you feeling helpless and without options. So do yourself a favor and find out what your legal options are. In the United States, start by visiting the Victim Rights Law Center website: www.victimrights.org, or call them directly at (617) 399-6720.

Dive In: Right now, whether or not you've ever experienced a sexual violation, go check out the websites of RAINN (www.rain.org) and the Victim Rights Law Center (www.victimrights.org). Learn about what they do, their philosophy, and the resources available on their websites. Spend at least fifteen minutes on each site. That way, if you ever find you need their services, you'll know where to turn.

SAFECALLS

If you're going out to meet someone you don't know very well and you think you might go somewhere private with them, I highly recommend setting up a "safecall." A safecall is a communication safety net you can build for yourself when you're not sure if the person you're going to be alone with is safe. It works like this:

1. Tell a friend what you're doing and whom you're doing it with. Be as specific as possible—full names, contact info, address of where you'll be if you have it.

2. Arrange a particular time to check in with your friend by phone. Be sure to agree on who's calling whom, so there's no confusion.

3. Decide whether or not you need a code. A phone call can go any number of ways. You certainly should say, "If I don't answer, and you don't hear from me, I'm in trouble." But you may also want to arrange a code in case you do pick up and want to tell your

friend that you're in trouble without alerting the person you're with that you're asking for help. Make it a specific word or phrase that will sound innocuous: "Things are super great" or "Did you remember to feed the cat?" This is especially important, depending on how you handle the next bit:

4. Decide whether or not you're going to tell your date you have a safecall. I like to let a date know, before I go back to their place, that I've set up a safecall. Just like the STD testing conversation from the last chapter, not only does this serve the practical purpose of letting a potential assailant know that they're unlikely to get away without consequences, but it also provides you with insight into their character, based on their reaction. Do they mock you? Are they defensive? Or are they accepting and understanding, saying some version of "Good for you; that's great you're taking care of yourself"? If I get a bad response to letting my date know about the safecall, I can bail before I even get to their house. And if I get a supportive response (as I do most of the time), it adds to my ability to trust this person, which can make the night go even better.

5. Agree on what should happen if you sound the alarm. If you don't pick up or call in at the arranged time, or if you give the code for "please send help," what do you want your friend to do? Contacting the authorities is the most popular option, but not all neighborhoods have equally responsive, upstanding enforcement officers. So use your judgment based on what you know of your local law enforcement department. Other options may include having

friends come get you. In extreme cases, of course,
that may put your friends in harm's way. There's
no perfect answer here, but it's in your and your
friends' best interests to pick your preferred one
long before it becomes necessary.

That's pretty much all there is to it. So, say you're going home
with someone you just met at a party. You might say to your
friend, "I'm going home with so-and-so. Here's their name and
the address where we're going. Will you call me in an hour to
check in?" Or you might say, "I'm going to meet someone I've
met online. We're meeting at this bar but might go back to their
place afterward. I'll text you with the address if I do that. If I
don't call you by eleven, please call me."

Ideally, talk with your friends about safecalls in advance,
so if you need to arrange for one on the spot, you'll know both
what the code is and what you want your friend to do if you
need help.

> **Dive In:** If you think you might ever want or
> need to use a safecall, reach out to a friend this week and
> ask them if they'll be your safecall partner. Talk through all
> the questions above, and when you've agreed on a plan
> that works for both of you, write it up and email it to them,
> and ask them to write back acknowledging that they've
> gotten it and agree to it, so that you'll both have it on
> hand for future reference. Maybe even put it on a little
> piece of paper in your wallet, with your friend's number,
> in case you can't access your own phone. (If you've got
> a smartphone, there may even be an app that facilitates

safecalls, like the Date Tracker Alert app for iPhone. You just input the time, location, and other details of your date into the app, along with a time by which you have to check in with the app. If you don't check in by that time, it sends out an alert to your designated emergency contacts.)

If you don't think you'll ever need or want a safecall for yourself, reach out to a friend who might want one of their own, and offer to be their safecall partner. Follow all the steps above.

 Go Deeper:

1. Try a different kind of safeword. The sexual safewords we discussed in this chapter serve as an efficient emergency brake for when you need to stop the action in bed. But they work just as well outside the bedroom, especially if you tend to get emotionally triggered to the point where it becomes difficult to explain to your partner when you need some special support or attention. If that's you, try arranging a separate safeword with your partner. Just pick a word that you can both remember and agree on (as with sexual safewords, it's best if you pick something that won't likely come up in conversation, like "rutabaga" or "platypus"), and agree on what it means if you say it. (Maybe it means you need a ten-minute timeout from whatever conversation you're having at the time, or maybe it means you need your partner, if possible, to drop everything else and turn all their attention to just holding you. You decide.)

These next exercises are designed to give your body a voice and to start a conversation between your physical, emotional, spiritual, and rational "selves." Of course, they are all one. I'm separating them out here because our *culture* has separated them out.

2. Write a letter of protest from your body to your brain. Does she *like* sitting in that chair all day tapping on a keyboard? I thought not! Wouldn't she be a *great* erotic dancer, given the chance (maybe even just solo in your bedroom in front of the mirror)? Why do you never let her *play*? Why all these darn rules about what she can ingest, how she should look and behave? All this judgment about the size of her tits and the shape of her bum? Why *can't* she have sex with that barista at Starbucks? For Goddess's sake—how do you think that makes her *feel* . . . ?

    She has a list of demands. (Write the list out.)

    End your letter with a one-sentence take-home message from your body to your self. Commit to meeting at least one item on your body's list of demands.

3. Draw a wellness wheel (see below).[2]

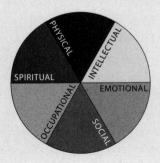

For one week, keep a record of how much and how long you operate in each slice of the pie. It might be hard to separate them out—for instance, a social activity (like taking a long walk or hike with friends) might also be intellectual, physical, and emotional.

At the end of the week, you might want to make some commitments—to get out more, go for a daily walk, or get back into yoga. And yes. This has *everything* to do with sex.

CHAPTER 9

DO UNTO OTHERS

THIS MAY BE A BOOK ABOUT FINDING OUT HOW TO HAVE a sexual life that's safe and satisfying for *you,* but if you're being sexual with another person, you also have a responsibility to do right by them—emotionally and physically. This can be a hard balance to strike. For many women, we've been taught our whole lives to put others' needs before our own, sometimes in ways that have caused us real harm over the years. But once we become aware of that dynamic, we can be tempted to overcompensate, focusing only on our needs, desires, and boundaries, to the exclusion of our partners'. Looking out for our partners can start to feel fraught and even dangerous to our sense of self. It's not always easy to know how to balance taking care of ourselves and asserting our own needs and desires with our responsibility toward our partners. And what about when we mess up and hurt ourselves or someone else?

You likely already know that it's not okay to deliberately violate someone's sexual boundaries or otherwise be emotionally or physically abusive to them. But there are also lots of ways we may hurt others inadvertently, just by being careless with our partners' needs and boundaries, being confused about our own motives, or tricking ourselves into thinking that we mean well when we're actually just putting off telling our partners difficult truths (which will inevitably hurt even more when they come out later). If we deserve partners who take care with our bodies and our feelings (and we do! Even you!), then we owe our partners the same consideration as well.

The Golden Rule is golden for a reason. If you do unto others as you would have them do unto you, you'll do right by both of you most of the time.

WHEN YOU AND YOUR PARTNER WANT DIFFERENT THINGS

It can be hard when you and your sexual partner don't want the same thing, especially when it's a relationship that's connected on levels other than physical. If it's a purely physical relationship and you're mismatched, it's probably best for everyone just to move on to a partner who better meets your needs. But if you're emotionally attached to each other, breaking up isn't the option most people want to consider first.

Often, incompatibility has to do with differences in libido, or how frequently each partner wants to have sex, but that's not the only way we can be sexually off with our partners. Maybe one of you likes it rough and fast and the other likes it soft and slow. Maybe you're not into each other's kinks. When Enoch went through a period of low sexual desire, ze[1] discovered that sex meant really different things to hir:

Physical intimacy, for my partner, was one of the major ways that we demonstrated our emotional closeness. So when that left, my partner felt like, I don't feel secure in your feelings for me. And that was hard. For me it was like, we have this wonderful relationship, and here's another part of it. And for her it was like, we have this wonderful relationship, and here's the most important expression of it.

Whatever your mismatch, there are a number of things you can do to try to bridge it, some points to keep in mind, and a few things you should most certainly *not* do, including the following:

Don't make it personal

Let's say you want to have sex with your partner every morning. You wake up feeling frisky, and there's your lover, looking sooo warm and desirable. It's an awesome feeling, isn't it? Uh . . . not so much when the feeling's not mutual. You get the equivalent of a swift kick in the shin and a "let me sleep already" grumble. Ouch.

Whether you're the one who wants "more" or "less" than your partner, it can feel frustrating, confusing, and downright personal—even when it's not. Like a referendum on your desirability or your worth. You will likely feel rejected, and it can also trigger insecurity about the characteristics you're most sensitive about: appearance, social skills, how your partner feels about your race or age, or whatever issue makes you feel vulnerable.

Whatever your mismatch is, it's not about you—any more than your desires are all about this person. Your desires are a reflection of your own sexuality, coupled with how a particular person makes you feel. And the same applies in reverse. Say you are desperately attracted to the outspoken tattooed girl in your class, but no amount of flirting or chatting or "accidental" brushes against her arm elicits even the slightest interest from her. Or, worse, you muster the courage to ask her out, and she says no without any hesitation. Even worse, she goes further and says it's because *she's simply not attracted to you.* It doesn't mean you're not attractive. Even if you're hot for someone and they're cold for you, it doesn't mean you're not smoking. All it means is that you don't light that particular person's fire. Even if they try to make it about you in some awful way—they tell you it's your race or age or size or sexual experience or sexual identity or income or anything else that feels like a criticism. That's a statement about them, *not* about you.

The same holds true on the flip side. Back to libido imbalance, as an example: There's nothing wrong with you if you're the person who's saying "no" or "not that" when it comes to sex. It doesn't make you "frigid" or "withholding" or "selfish" or "uptight" or whatever. And it doesn't mean your partner's desires are wrong, either. It just means your desires are different from your partner's.

Don't make assumptions

Sometimes we mistakenly make assumptions about our partners' sexual behavior. For example, many women (and some men) assume that men want sex all the time. That they'll never say no to sex, especially with a woman they were hot for to begin with.

Big fallacy.

I'll tell you a little secret: Men are not pneumatic drills. Some men have a much stronger sex drive than other men, and even those men with a strong sex drive have moods and phases and health issues and stress and all manner of things that are (sing it with me!) *not about you* that may impact their desire to be sexual with you. So don't assume that if your partner is male, he's always going to want more sex than you. Assuming your relationship is going well, a guy's not wanting you when you want him probably means he's simply not in the mood.

Similarly, don't buy into the stereotype that a person of color is going to want more sex than a white person, or that a woman with a trauma history wants kinkier sex than you do because she's damaged (or that she's turning you down because she's too fragile), etc.

If you want to find out more about your partner's sexual desires and limits, get to a place where you're genuinely curious about and open to hearing what they have to say, and then ask them.

Don't apply pressure

What if you believe the person you desire just needs a little convincing to see things your way sexually? You may even feel compelled to try to convince them how awesome sex could be if they did it *your* way, or maybe you can talk them out of whatever's holding them back. Like, "You know, baby, anal sex isn't *that* painful, if you just relax . . . " Or, "I know you're tired, but if you just lie back and let me touch you, I can make you want me."

The problem with this approach is the assumption that your desire to have sex (or a certain kind of sex) is more important than their desire *not* to. When it comes to partnered sex, it really does take two to tango, and so everyone has veto power. You have to respect that. And not just respect it if you can't convince them to change their mind—*really* respect it.

Why? Well, aside from being the right thing to do, and one of the easiest ways to avoid sexually assaulting someone, it's also a good way to get where you want to be. You want your partner to be hot for you? To take risks with you? To be vulnerable with you? Then they need to know they can trust you. They need to feel like they're choosing to play with you of their own free will. They need the space to get clear about what they really really want, so that they can be freely sexy with you. You've got to back off if they say "no," or even if they say "not right now."

So what can you do? Well, for one, talk and listen. Did you notice I didn't say just "talk"? Too often, when we are having issues with our partners, we forget that simply talking at our partner won't solve anything. Instead, be genuinely curious about their point of view. Ask them questions and invite them to share their perspective. And not with the goal of changing their mind or pointing out that they're wrong—with the goal of empathizing, understanding and really absorbing where they're coming from. One of the coolest things about being in any kind of relationship—whether it be sexual or not—is the chance to see the world through someone else's eyes. It expands the realm of what we can imagine as possible.

Don't get me wrong—this can be difficult. When sex and feelings are on the line, things can feel heated. Like you won't be able to breathe until you can get your partner to agree with you or see it your way. You go into the conversation looking for chinks in their armor, holes in their argument, any opening for you to wedge yourself into. It can feel really awesome! You made your partner see things your way! You changed their mind! You're powerful!

Except . . .

Over time, this dynamic will eat away at the trust in your relationship. Your partner will feel like they're always battling with you. And you know what's not a warm or sexy feeling? Feeling defensive all the time.

On the flip side, the talking-and-listening approach works only if your partner is doing the same thing for you. Do they genuinely want to know and understand your point of view so that you can be a better team? Or do they often discount your opinions and tell you all about why you're wrong and they're right? If it's the latter, you may have larger problems than mismatched sexual desires. If it's the former, then you have a strong base in place to help you work through this challenge.

Once you've really talked and listened to each other about the issue (for some ideas about how to do active listening exchanges with your partner, check out the resources at www .wyrrw.com/activelistening), you've got to deal with the tricky part. Because understanding and even empathizing with each other's positions is essential, but it's probably not going to solve the problem on its own. Unless that listening process has revealed an obvious solution that's easy for you both, you're going to now have to negotiate a compromise. And compromising about sex can be difficult. Up until now, we've focused on not settling for less than what you really really want. But when it comes to compromise, the phrase takes on a new meaning. You have to decide: What is it that you really *really* want, and what is it that you want that's less important and possible to sacrifice in order to meet your partner halfway? This may take some time and experimentation. Don't expect to come to an agreement right away, and even when you do come to one, it's a great idea to check in and see how the arrangement is working for you both, so you can make adjustments as necessary.

The other tough truth is this: It may not be possible to find a compromise that's healthy for both of you. You may genuinely be sexually incompatible. Sometimes this is temporary— work stress, health issues, emotional difficulties, even just the plain old up and downs of life can all affect our sexual desires, and you're not always going to shift in sync with your partners. If you're invested in the relationship, you may want to give it some time to see if and how things evolve. But sometimes sexual incompatibility goes beyond being temporary. And compromise isn't always the answer.

Becca puts it best. "When talking about a disagreement, compromise can be a good thing. But when talking about yourself, it's more like a bridge. If a bridge is compromised, you don't want to go over it. Coming to a compromise with someone else is really different than compromising yourself."

In other words, meeting your partner somewhere in the middle is great, as long as you can both feel pretty whole there. But if you're compromising a central part of yourself in order to compromise with your partner about sex, that's dangerous for both of you. It may be hard to tell the difference sometimes. It can even be useful to check in with a trusted friend or therapist as you negotiate these waters. But ultimately, only you can know when your compromise is building a bridge that strengthens your relationship or tearing down something structurally important inside you.

Dive In: Make a list of compromises you've made with sexual partners. Maybe one of you agreed to try something new or initiate sex more—or less. Maybe one of you wanted sex in the context of a more committed relationship than the other one was offering, and you had sex anyhow. Write down the compromises you explicitly made and discussed with your partner, as well as the ones you decided you were willing to make without talking about it. Include ones that worked out well and ones that felt awful or went badly. List as many as you can think of. If you don't have many, list compromises you've made with friends and family about nonsexual things, too. You should make sure to have at least ten compromises on your list, though if you've got more, list 'em all!

Now, make two columns on a page in your notebook. Label them "Building" and "Breaking." Using the list you just generated, move all the compromises that helped build a stronger connection with your partner to the "Building" column, and all the compromises that harmed or broke something inside you to the "Breaking" column. Put a star next to any of the compromises that go in both columns.

> Now look at the two columns. What do the "Building" compromises have in common? What kinds of compromises are they? What influenced your decision to make those compromises, and how did you feel about them before and during the decision to compromise? What about the "Breaking" compromises? Is there anything that's true, generally, about the compromises in one column but not about the other? If you can't find any patterns yourself, ask a friend to look at your list with you. The point of these lists is to help you tell helpful from hurtful the next time you're faced with a choice about compromising.

LYING

No one needs to be told that it's immoral to lie in order to get what you want sexually. In theory, we all know it's wrong to lie. In practice, it's a little messier. Because as we grow up, we learn that there all kinds of circumstances in which it's actually okay to lie, or when it's even considered polite or kind. We learn to say, "I mailed it yesterday" as we're scrambling to the post office. We tell our old coworker how happy we are to see her when we run into her at the grocery store, even though "never seeing her again" was high on our list of things to celebrate when we left that job. And so we get used to the idea that actually, some lies are okay. If no one finds out, no one gets hurt.

However, when coupled with sex, lying becomes more complicated. If your partner doesn't have all the relevant information, they can't enthusiastically consent to what's going on. And that means lying can lead to some serious boundary violations.

But what's "all the relevant information"? And how much is it your responsibility to offer it?

Let's do the easy part first. If your partner asks you a question that's relevant to your sexual interactions and you actively lie—that is, you give an answer you know to be untrue—in addition to proving yourself untrustworthy, you have absolutely voided their ability to enthusiastically consent. So if your partner asks if you have any STDs, and you do but you say that you don't? That's straight-up bad. Same goes if your partner asks if you're cool with this relationship being casual and you say yes, even though you really want something deeper or longer-lasting. And if you offer false information without even being asked . . . ? Yeah. You get the idea. Just as you deserve to know the truth of the situation, so does your partner. Without truthful communication, your partner can't make good decisions about what they do and don't want to do with you sexually.

The "no lying" rule applies to emotional manipulation as well. If you invent a crisis, exaggerate your feelings, withhold affection, deliberately flirt with other people in front of your partner when you know that gets them jealous, or basically do anything devious in order to get a particular kind of attention from your partner? That's lying, too, and it's only going to create mistrust and hurt between you in the long run.

(There are some caveats here. If you're lying to your partner because you fear for your safety by telling the truth, that's different. If your partner asks if they look good, and you know they put some effort into looking attractive for you, even though you really hate that color on them? Lying can be kind in that situation, too.)

But what about lies of omission? What about the stuff you don't say that you're pretty sure your partner really would care about if they knew, that might even endanger their safety, but that you'd just as soon not say because you'd be less likely to get what you want?

The most obvious example of this is cheating. Simply put: It's not nice to cheat. (Yes, duh.) Unless there are extenuating circumstances (your partner is in a coma), if you find yourself irresistibly drawn to someone else while you're in a monogamous relationship, you really have to 'fess up. Your partner deserves to know ahead of time that you no longer want to be in a monogamous relationship, so that they can make decisions of their own. This is never easy. You may not want to lose them, and you may want to avoid hurting them. You may have children together, and you don't want to risk breaking up your family. But telling before succumbing to temptation really is the decent thing to do. If you don't, you're voiding your partner's ability to enthusiastically consent to the terms of your relationship (which will no longer be as they seem). Beyond that, if you know you're being untrustworthy and your partner doesn't, you'll begin to wonder if your partner is doing the same to you. All this does is undermine the agreements on which your relationship is built, and with them, any trust or intimacy between you.

Even if you're not thinking of cheating, another very common lie of omission is simply neglecting to tell someone you're not into them. Whether your feelings have changed or were never there in the first place, you may think you're doing them a favor by "not hurting them." Unless there's a specific, short-term reason to hold off delivering the bad news (they're studying for their finals, they're about to have surgery, etc.), the only person you're favoring is yourself—by avoiding guilt over hurting them. Ultimately, you're putting off the inevitable, and in the meantime, you may be sending your erstwhile paramour some very confusing (and possibly hurtful) mixed signals, all the while building up stress and anxiety for yourself and short-changing your own needs to avoid potential hurt feelings. A terrible, toxic cocktail. Don't drink it.

There are other examples of omissions, however, that are much less clear. You can't be expected to know everything your partner wants to know in order to consent to sex. Here I'm talking about things like your sexual history, or whether or not you're sexually involved with anyone else at the moment. It could also be your gender or sexual identity, or your political or religious beliefs, or how much money you make, or how old you are. These are all things that some people may care about and some people may not, but it's on them to ask if they want to know.

When deciding when to withhold true information, the Buddhists have a more positive spin on the question, a useful idea called "wise speech." In order to be considered "wise speech," something must be not just true, but also kind and helpful. If you're omitting something true because it would be both unkind and unhelpful, you're probably doing the right thing. For example, not telling your partner that his voice grates on your nerves sometimes is a good omission, as, since he can't do anything

about the sound of his voice, telling him would clearly be both
unkind and unhelpful. If something is true and helpful but not
kind, like the bad kissing we discussed in chapter 8, you've got
to balance how helpful it might be (to you and them) against
how unkind it is.

> **Dive In:** Make a list of every lie you can
> remember ever telling a sexual partner. Include the whop-
> pers as well as the white lies—"I love you" (when it wasn't
> true) as well as "you look great today." Include lies of omis-
> sion, too, especially the ones you omitted deliberately.
> (That is, you thought about telling someone something
> that might have impacted your relationship, and then
> decided against it.) Include lies you got busted for telling
> and lies that have never been found out, even to this day.
>
> Now, cross out every lie about which you believe the
> recipient of the lie would agree with you that it was kind
> of you to tell. Then cross out every lie of omission that
> you omitted because it really, genuinely wasn't any of your
> partner's business.
>
> What lies are you left with? Do they form a pattern of
> any kind? What do you tend to lie about, and what moti-
> vates you to lie? How do those lies tend to turn out? How
> do they make you feel?

WOMAN UP

As you surely know by now, there are a lot of challenging things about being female and sexual. So it can feel tempting to some of us to take advantage of the few privileges it affords us, especially if our partners are men or masculine-identified. And that's all well and good if you and your partner are both into it and the privileges are symbolic: door-opening, dinner-buying kind of privileges. (Though even there, it's not a bad idea to check in to see if your partner enjoys these gestures or feels obligated to do them.)

But there are other kinds of sexual advantages that can come with your womanhood that I encourage you to do your best to reject, such as letting your partner make the first move— or all the moves. Why do I suggest that you give up that position of luxury? Because it may well suck for your partner. They may not want to have to do all the work and take on all the risk. And even if they don't mind, it can keep you passive about your desires and instead make you a screen onto which your partner's desires are projected.

Of course, whether or not you're expected to make the first move depends on characteristics beyond being female. What are the sexual proclivities of the people you're sleeping with? Do others see you as more masculine, feminine, genderqueer, androgynous?

Avory, who identifies as genderqueer, knows all about this dynamic:

I look fairly butch (if you want to use those words), and I identify as submissive. And both of my girlfriends identify very strongly as tops or dominant, but very femme, and very girlie. When we met, both of them were so sweet and shy, and nobody was initiating anything. I feel uncomfortable initiating, but once I gave the slightest little indication, like, okay, I'm interested in you, then their dominant attitude took over. But they were so socialized into being girlie, that starting wasn't something they could do.

If you're the type of woman who's been socially conditioned to be sexually passive, it's so very tempting to let your partner make all the moves. It's so much less emotionally risky than taking the initiative yourself. Not to mention all the stigmas that can come with being perceived as a "sexually aggressive" woman, a label that's slapped on most of us if we dare to become actors on behalf of our own desires.

But if you don't try to make things happen for yourself at least some of the time, you're telling both yourself and your partner that you're a passenger on this ride, and not a pilot. That's going to make it much harder when it comes to getting what you really really want. It's also incredibly inconsiderate to your partner, who in all likelihood is just as nervous as you and will eventually grow to resent having to do all the heavy lifting.

Think about it another way: Women are often expected to do the emotional work in a relationship. Do you ever tire of being the one who has to bring up emotional issues? Wish your partner would initiate those conversations some of the time?

Well, if you let your partner initiate all the sex, they're going to wind up feeling the same way about you. And that's not going to be sexy for either of you.

(A caveat applies here: If you're in a sexual partnership with someone who genuinely likes being the sexual aggressor, and it makes you both hot to have one of you always be in charge of starting things and the other always responding, by all means, have at it! But don't assume that's true without checking with your partner first.)

> **Dive In:** Write a sex scene in which you make all the moves. How do you initiate a first kiss? How do you try to turn up the heat while practicing enthusiastic consent? How do you respond if your partner needs you to slow down or doesn't want to do something in particular? What if you start doing something that you think will be hot, but you find out you don't like it? Add some of these elements into your scene, especially if they worry you. But don't forget to make it hot and fun for everyone involved. Give yourselves a happy ending!

FETISHIZING

We've already talked about what it feels like to be fetishized or "othered" by a partner. But it's worth saying directly how important it is to avoid doing this to someone else. Attraction is a funny and fickle thing—you may be attracted to someone for any number of random or specific reasons. You may have a "type" (in terms of appearance or personality), or you may not.

But there's a difference between finding caramel-colored skin hot and having that be the consistent deciding factor for whom you'll want to get with and whom you'll reject.

There are three main components to fetishizing, and so there are three levels to making sure you're not doing it. First and foremost, you'll want to check your intentions. Are you reducing your lust objects to one or two defining characteristics, or is there an interactive combination platter of factors that mix and match to spark an attraction? (In other words: Is that caramel skin all it takes, regardless of any other characteristics? Or is it the skin mixed with their nerdy *Doctor Who* obsession mixed with the way they dress or their taste in music that lights your fire?) And while you're checking in, ask yourself further: Is it the characteristic itself that makes you hot, or what it represents (that you're "hip" or "open-minded" for dating this person, that their "hot-bloodedness" reflects well on your ability to satisfy in bed, etc.)? Is it about the two of you getting together in private, or is it more about being able to tell your friends about it later?

Once you've got your internal motives clear, you still need to check in about your behavior. You're going to want to be extra careful in expressing your attraction to characteristics that may have left your partner vulnerable to discrimination or oppression. So if you're attracted to ample-size lovers, be careful not to overgeneralize (don't suggest that all fat people are hot, for example, because then your mate might think they're merely a fetish to you). Instead, be sure to also compliment the other attributes of theirs that you find attractive.

Which brings us to the third way to ensure you're not fetishizing your partner: Find out how they're feeling! You may have the best of intentions and be incredibly thoughtful about your behavior, but if it's not making your partner feel wanted for the right reasons, that really matters. (It doesn't mean you're necessarily doing something "wrong;" it just means whatever dynamic is going down between you isn't making your partner feel hot.)

So how can you tell whether your partner's feeling fetishized? The best way to find out is to simply *ask*. That may feel a little awkward, but isn't it better than inadvertently hurting your partner? Use the communication strategies from chapter 7, and check in with them. Tell your partner you recognize that they may have some history of feeling fetishized for the characteristic you're attracted to, and you want make sure you're not playing into that. Then shut up and listen. And if there are some hurt feelings, find out what, if anything, you can do differently to avoid causing them in the future.

Dive In: Go back to the list of partner preferences you developed in chapter 6. Are there any characteristics that attract you to a partner that your partner may have had fetishized about them in the past? Spend ten minutes writing about what it is about those characteristics that turns you on, and what strategies you can (or already do!) employ to make sure your partner knows you're hot for them for the right reasons.

SHAME

It may seem pretty obvious to say, "Don't shame your partner!" But actually avoiding doing it is another thing altogether.

As we've explored in earlier chapters, we're all taught to feel shame about any number of things related to our sexuality: our desires, our boundaries, our bodies, our wardrobes, the kinds of people we're attracted to . . . By now you know, at least intellectually, that as long as you're not hurting yourself or anyone else, there's nothing to be ashamed of when it comes to sex. But knowing it and feeling it are two different things.

Think back to that stereo equalizer. If you've learned sexual shame from one source or another, it's hard to ever get rid of it entirely. The best you can do is tone it way down. Unfortunately, that leaves open the possibility that you may inadvertently project your shame onto your partner in one way or another. Maybe you feel constantly vigilant about your body and whether it's attractive, and your partner doesn't seem nearly as invested, and this sparks feelings of resentment in you. Maybe one of you has a high sex drive and the other not so much, and you see your partner's difference as an abnormality. On the other hand, maybe you've successfully minimized some of your hang-ups—about your sexual fantasies or kinks, for example—but your partner still seems really, well, hung up. Or maybe you feel insecure about your boundaries—you get sexual with someone only when you're in a committed, monogamous relationship, maybe, and your partner has no such limit, and it makes you feel inadequate or unsure of yourself.

In any of these situations, you're at risk of encouraging your partner to feel ashamed, even if you don't mean to. Whether it's jealousy (you've been a "good girl," and your partner seems to feel free to ignore social norms), fear (your partner is willing to take risks that you never would), or judgment (you think you're more "evolved" than your partner), if you're not aware of the feelings that the differences between you and your partner inspire, they're likely to come out sideways and encourage your partner to feel bad.

So pay attention. If you notice that there's tension between your approaches to sexuality, spend some time getting in tune with yourself about how it makes you feel. And if you find you're judging yourself or your partner, it's time to come clean. Odds are, your partner may have some concerns of their own. If you share them in a way that takes responsibility, it can be something the two of you work on together, instead of a wedge of bad feeling pushing you apart. What you say can be as simple as, "I know I'm having these feelings, and they're not fair or rational, and I'm doing my best not to take them out on you. Can you help me resist them?" And then, as in all challenging conversations, shut up and actively listen.

Dive In: Reread your sexual mission statement from chapter 2. Do you still agree with it? Edit it in any way you see fit. Then write for ten minutes about the parts of the mission statement that are hardest for you to apply to yourself or a partner. Where do you get hung up? What shame are you having trouble letting go of?

MAKING AMENDS

Chances are, if you've been sexual with people before, then you've hurt people before, either emotionally or physically or both. That's to be expected—it's impossible to be intimate with people without occasionally bumping up against them in painful ways. We all say the wrong thing sometimes, or we're unintentionally selfish, insensitive, or thoughtless, or we break someone's heart because our feelings and needs just don't match up well enough with theirs. We all hurt people we care about sometimes, even if we haven't done anything wrong.

But if you've done something that's *really* harmed someone else—especially something avoidable, like leading someone on, or cheating on them, or pressuring them into doing something sexually they didn't want to do—it's important to take stock of that and try to make amends with them and forgive yourself in the bargain. Accepting that you're human and fallible is important: Having hurt someone, even in a big way, doesn't make you evil or irredeemable. The Golden Rule applies here: If someone hurt you in an avoidable way, wouldn't you want them to at least try to make amends? Living up to that ideal yourself will not only help your partners but also reinforce that you deserve to be treated the way you treat others.

So. What are we really talking about here? Well, it depends on what you've done, how avoidable it was, and how much it's impacted your partner. Did you call them names? Did you cheat on them? Did you lead them on when you knew you weren't that interested in them? Did you give them an STD? Did you violate their sexual boundaries?

It can be uncomfortable to face up to these sorts of things. None of us want to think of ourselves as the kind of person who'd do something like that. These actions don't have to define you. But they will if you let them fester without attending to them.

Because, as it turns out, an apology is hardly ever unwelcome. (It's hardly ever enough, but that doesn't mean you shouldn't do it.) But don't apologize if you're not genuinely sorry, and don't give a nonapology apology. Don't say, "I'm sorry if your feelings were hurt" or any nonsense like that that attempts to downplay your responsibility. If you know you did wrong and you feel remorse, own it. Say, "Here's what I did wrong, and here's how I know it's affecting or affected you, and here's what I'm going to do to prevent myself from doing it again . . . and please know that I take full responsibility and I'm truly sorry." Do it even if the harm you caused happened a long time ago. It's never too late to apologize, as long as you don't expect the apology to make it all better.

After you've apologized and listened carefully to their response, ask yourself this question: Does this person need any immediate or long-term help as a result of my actions? If, say, you gave them herpes, do they need medical care that you can pay for? Or, if you can't afford to pay for it, can you help them find a free health clinic? Do they need mental health services? Or housing if, say, they had to move out because you did something that made them no longer feel safe around you? Taking practical responsibility for your actions can go a long way.

For Heather, age forty-one, making amends was a long and complex process.

My current partner is actually someone I was with over twenty years ago. The relationship ended the first time because I was suddenly dealing with PTSD from previous sexual assaults that I was unprepared to deal with and dealt with incredibly badly. Some of dealing with it badly involved basically abandoning my partner and shutting him out completely.

A bunch of years after that, we reconnected so I could apologize and take responsibility for the emotional harm I caused. It was horribly painful, and it was also tricky to do because my partner obviously did not hold me responsible for the assaults that caused my PTSD. It was very important to me that I was still understood as responsible for how I reacted to it.

Then, many years after that we reconnected and pursued a relationship again, and in doing so still both had some baggage from before to unpack. Again, it wasn't easy, but one thing I did was to facilitate a counseling session for us to get some help in working that out together, which was both an excellent help and very clearly understood as a strong commitment from me to really work through the damage from before.

The help your partner needs may be more abstract. Maybe they need a friend, or a hug, or general emotional support. But if they tell you there's nothing you can do, or to simply leave them alone, then abiding by that is the best way to "make it up" to them. Pushing this hurt person to let you do some active demonstration of penance when they want no part of it is about your wanting to feel better about yourself—it's not a way to make amends to someone you've hurt.

There may also be consequences to you. You may lose your relationship with the person you've hurt. Your friends may be angry with you. You may face legal trouble. Whatever the direct consequences to you, the best way to demonstrate your remorse is to accept them. Respect your partner's decision to leave. Apologize to your friends and accept their anger. Plead guilty to those legal charges if you're guilty. Own your actions, and their impact will go away faster than if you fight responsibility. And you'll have a greater chance of healing the damage you've done, to boot.

Once you've done everything you can to help ameliorate this damage, the last question to focus on is this: How is it that I came to do this hurtful thing to someone I care about, and how can I avoid doing it again? These are questions that only you can answer.

> **Dive In:** There's no better way to practice this than to just do it. Make a list of the things you most regret doing to a partner. Did you tell a lie, use deliberately hurtful words, blame or shame them for things that weren't their fault, violate a boundary? Whatever it is, it already happened. Don't use this list to beat yourself up. Just pick one, reach out to the person you wronged, and sincerely and fully apologize. Then pay attention to whatever response you get and look for opportunities to make further amends. Don't go in assuming the person is still hurt or needs something specific from you—put them

in the driver's seat. Ask them how they feel or what they might or might not need. You may hope for forgiveness, but don't make that your goal.

If your list is troubling to you, spend some time writing about what it is that troubles you. Do you have unhealthy patterns of behavior? What motivates you to do these hurtful things? What strategies could you try to be less hurtful in the future? Be as honest as you can with yourself. You never have to show this to anyone.

Take a deep breath. This chapter may have been hard for you in new ways, and that's not surprising, nor does it make you a bad person. In fact, most people never take as much care in considering how they're treating their partners as you now have. And as a bonus, the more you clarify your values about how your partners deserve to be treated, the more you become the partner you think they deserve, the more you'll teach yourself that you deserve all of these things, too.

Go Deeper: Think of some people you'd like to tell something important to but can't. It might be that they are dead, or that they don't want to speak to you anymore (or you to them), or that they moved and you lost their address. It might even be that you met them only once and didn't even know their name, but somehow they said or did something that changed you, or you said or did something that may have changed them, for better or for worse.

Write them a letter, even though you know you can't send it.

These are the rules:

1. You must name, exactly, the behavior, incident, or relationship that occurred—tie it down if you can with dates and details.

2. You must name, exactly, the effect it had on you and/or that you imagine it had on them.

3. You must express the feeling or feelings you were left with—shame, joy, inspiration, guilt, anger, grief.

4. You must say how you imagine they felt afterward.

5. You must say why you are writing, and why you are writing now, rather than earlier or later.

6. You must say what you learned from your relationship with that person.

7. You must find something to thank them for.

8. You must make a wish.

9. You must describe the gift you are enclosing—don't worry if it can't be wrapped or mailed—think small or big, real or imaginary.

10. You must sign it with your full name.

CHAPTER 10

FRIENDS AND FAMILY

GIVEN ALL THE WORK YOU'VE DONE EXPLORING YOUR influences, you surely already know how powerful an impact your friends and family can have on your sex life. We've talked quite a bit about how to evaluate and turn the volume either up or down on those influences, but the reality is, when it comes to the people close to you, nothing is static. Often, we can't just say yes or no to the messages our loved ones are sending us—we have to engage with them about those messages, set boundaries, and encourage them to have healthier sexual attitudes.

You can also draw on your friends and family as a source of strength as you navigate your sexual relationships. If you have a history of getting blame, shame, and fear from your friends and family, it can be hard to see them as anything but a problem. But the truth is, if you're lucky and you play your cards right, your friends and family can be an incredible source of support and inspiration when it comes to developing a great relationship with your own sexuality.

Okay, maybe not all of them. Maybe your uncle will always be a creep and your childhood best friend will never stop judging your sexual choices. You can't change everyone. But you can develop friendships with people who share (or at least support) your sexual values, and in many cases, even if your family isn't the sex-positive dream you wish it was, you can still find allies within it who can make it easier to negotiate the ties that bind.

Surrounding yourself with supportive people is critical when it comes to building a healthy sexual life for yourself. One of the key ways to turn down the volume on the Terrible Trio and amplify the awesomeness of your authentic sexual voice is to spend as much time as you can with folks who model the attitudes toward sexuality you aspire to. These are the people who are going to cheer you on as you put yourself out there, build up your confidence when you succumb to doubt or shame, and take care of you when risks don't pay off. At those moments, don't you want people around you who understand that there is no pleasure or satisfaction without some kind of risk, who won't blame you for trying things but rather will remind you of how brave you were to do so, even if it doesn't always work out? Wouldn't you rather lean on folks who'll tell you that you deserve better if someone treats you badly, rather than those who'll suggest you "got what you deserved"?

And don't just think about what they *tell* you. We learn so much from the people we're closest to by watching how they behave toward others. If the people around you treat sexual women like trash, you're going to draw the logical conclusion that they'd think the same of you "if they only knew." (The reverse also holds true: If your friends are constantly trying to top each other's exploits and treat you like a child if you won't "compete," you're going to start to feel pressure to perform, whether you want to or not.)

Twenty-seven-year-old Idalia learned an even more challenging lesson this way.

Once I was old enough, my mom was very open with her own sexuality and the right of women to enjoy themselves. She joked about sex all the time. But at the same time, she was also in more than one emotionally abusive relationship, including one that lasted over ten years. I somehow connected one with the other, and it took me years before I could really open up sexually to myself and another person, without being terrified that I would end up caged and losing my independence like I saw happen around me as a child. I couldn't explore my sexuality until I learned to trust that I knew the difference between love/ affection and manipulation.

It's true that you can't choose your family. And you may not want to cut yourself off from old friends, even if you recognize that they're sending you messages that aren't good for your sexual sanity. But you can certainly give special appreciation to those in your life who support your healthy sexuality, and be choosy when it comes to making new friends. And there are definitely things you can do to improve some of the challenging relationships you may already have.

Of course, all good relationships go both ways. That means
that the Golden Rule applies in this chapter as well: Be the
friend you want your friends to be to you. Be as loving and
open toward your mother as you want her to be to you. It's not
that complicated, especially given how far you've come through
this book. All it means is that you need to pay attention. Are
you projecting your sexual values onto people who don't share
them? Are you assuming all your friends aspire to your level of
sexual experience, or that they all want sex to be as emotionally intimate and special as you do? Are you scandalized by
your mother's new girlfriend because you can't handle thinking of your mom as a sexual person who gets to make her own
choices? Do you insist on snuggling your nieces and nephews
regardless of what they want? Do you go on and on about how
awesome your sexual values are without making room to listen
to other people? You can't expect to build relationships that
support what you really really want if you don't make room
for the people you're relating to to make different choices
for themselves.

> **Dive In:** Go back to chapter 2 and reread
> your sexual mission statement. Now that you've spent so
> much time exploring your sexual values and desires, you
> may find you want to add to it or edit it. Feel free to draw
> on any of the writing or lists you've done for other exer-
> cises in other chapters. Work on it as long as it takes to
> make it feel complete and true for you today.

FRIENDS IN LOW PLACES

Sometimes talking to friends and family about your sexual values is more for their benefit than for yours. Specifically, sometimes your friends or relations are going to find themselves entangled in sexual or romantic relationships that look unhealthy to you.

It can be tough to know how to approach these situations. On the one hand, you want to help the people you care about have happy, healthy lives, so when you see them in a situation that's making them unhappy and may be putting them at emotional or physical risk, the desire to intervene can be quite powerful. On the other hand, you want to be a supportive, nonjudgmental friend, and that sometimes means supporting decisions that you would never have made yourself.

To add to the complexity, it can be very difficult to really know what it's like inside someone else's relationship. Let's take it in the reverse first, because it's easier to see. Have you ever admired someone's relationship, thought they seemed like the perfect couple, only to find yourself shocked when they broke up, or when one or the other of them revealed how miserable they were? If this hasn't happened yet, I promise it will more than once in your life. "Perfect" couples don't exist—if a couple seem like they have no problems at all, I guarantee you they're either (a) a completely brand-new couple or (b) covering up a more complex reality.

Do your friends a favor and don't ever put them on the "perfect couple" pedestal. You may mean it as high praise— even if it's tinged with envy—but it's a trap for your pals, who now will be reluctant to tell you anything that tarnishes the image you have of them. And a couple who can't talk with their friends about their problems is a couple that's ultimately going to run into trouble. Though it may seem counterintuitive, telling a couple they're perfect is the opposite of support: It's pressure.

As ill-advised as it can be to tell your friend their relationship is perfect, it's much harder to know what to do when you think the opposite of them. So before you plow ahead and stick your nose where it's not helpful, consider the following:

Mismatch or Mistreatment?

What, exactly, is bothering you about your friends' relationship? Do you think they're just not suited for each other in the long term? Perhaps you think your friend could do better, or maybe you simply don't like their companion, but you have no evidence that your friend is unhappy? These situations can be awkward, but it's best to keep your opinion to yourself unless you're asked directly. And if your friend does ask your thoughts on their partner and those thoughts are less than rosy? Tread carefully. Once you tell your best friend their lover is beneath them, you can't unsay that. Not only are you insulting their taste, but it's going to make things awkward if they get married. Try something more neutral but truthful, like, "Your sweetie's not my cup of tea, but you seem happy. Are you?" Even if they say they're having doubts, let them lead the conversation, and don't pile on. If you bash their beloved because it seems like they're heading for a breakup anyhow, they're going to remember that if they get back together with the person. A good, basic guideline is this: Never say anything stronger than they're saying.

On the other hand, if you think your friend is being (or has been) mistreated, that's another matter. (We'll talk about whether you think your friend is the one doing the mistreating in a minute.) If you think your friend is being physically or emotionally abused by their partner, you're going to want to reach out—but do it carefully.

Take a peek back at chapter 5 to review some common signs of relationship abuse. If you notice any of these red flags, or other signs that trouble you, the first thing to do is ask yourself this question: Does my friend seem to see these signs, too? Do they seem to want help, or will they resist my efforts?

You're asking this because it's tricky helping someone who doesn't want help, and it takes a very delicate approach. Especially if you're trying to help someone who's being mistreated in a relationship.

Think about that list. What is the one thing all of those symptoms have in common? Whether it's emotional or physical abuse, the abusive partner spends a lot of time trying to make their victim feel helpless so that they will rely on the abuser more and more, and thus be more easily manipulated. That's what makes this situation so tricky—often the victim is convinced they have no better options, that they're lucky to be with the abuser. From the outside, that can seem mystifying. But it's crucial to remember, because if you swoop in and tell them they're in a bad relationship and they need to get out, how do you think they're going to feel? Probably like someone else is telling them, yet again, what they should do with their life and their body. It may seem strange to you, since you have their well-being at heart and the abuser obviously doesn't, but you're going to seem very similar to the abuser, because you're suggesting that you know better than they what they should do.

On the other hand, if you show them that you have faith in their ability to think and act on their own behalf, you may actually be able to reach them. Start by asking them how they think the relationship is going, and really listen. Do they express fears or reservations about some of the dynamics between them and their partner? If so, steer the conversation in that direction; give them lots of room to explore and express those feelings.

If they claim all's well but you think they're in a dangerous or unhealthy situation, you're going to have to broach the subject. Remember, don't tell them what you think they should do. Instead, tell them that you're noticing behavior that concerns you. Be specific—give examples of the behavior that concerns you (for example, they've dropped off the map and won't return your calls, or you've seen their partner verbally tear them down). Always explain as clearly as you can *why* it worries you. Perhaps give examples of relationships you know of with healthier dynamics, as an example of how things can be different. Then ask them what they think of the relationship you've just described. Try not to argue with them. Really listen and understand. If they're excusing away dangerous behavior, having you tell them that they're wrong isn't going to help. Instead, tell them you're glad they're happy, but your concerns remain. Then emphasize that whether or not they need you right now, you're always there for them. One of the main ways abusers instill helplessness and vulnerability in their victims is by isolating them from their friends. Don't play into this dynamic—be sure they know you're not going anywhere, no matter what they do or don't do.

Remember, too, that you may be giving them advice that conflicts with what their partner is telling them, or with advice they're getting from other friends and family. Mieko ran up against this when trying to help a friend who was being mistreated by an ex:

Her parents' views on the situation and how she was allowed to feel and react to it were a lot different than what I felt, which was, It's okay to be angry, it's okay to be upset, if you feel like they treated you wrong you should tell them, and if you feel like you need space from them, you should be okay to take that space. *But her parents and some of her other friends were like, "Well, you know, you should forgive him immediately. Don't be so selfish."*

If you feel like a lone voice in the wilderness and you want to strengthen your case to your friend, don't get louder or more insistent. Instead, offer them resources that seem credible to back up your point of view—resources like this book, or *Our Bodies, Ourselves,* the website Scarleteen, or a community leader who your friend will trust and who is empathetic to your cause. There are many organizations working against relationship violence that offer lists of how to tell you're being mistreated and other resources.

Here's where it gets frustrating. You've tried to help, and they've refused. The terrible truth is that you can't help someone who doesn't want help. All you can do is let them know that they have options and support. When it comes to people we love who are being abused, it can be difficult to swallow, but it's still true. And that's why, if you're in this situation, the other thing to do is get support for yourself. Talk to friends and family about it. You can also call whatever hotlines in your area are available to support rape or abuse victims to get guidance on how you can help them.

(If you can't find anything near you, and you're in the United States, call RAINN—the Rape, Abuse & Incest National Network. Their national hotline is at (800) 656-HOPE. They also run an online hotline, which can be accessed wherever you are in the world, as long as you have an Internet connection: www.rainn.org.)

Once you've done all you can and you're feeling like you've got all the support you need, the only other thing you can do is to make good on your promise and be there for your friend no matter what. Check in with them once in a while, but don't be too pushy—don't make your concern for them the subject of conversation every single time you hang out. Just be their friend. Refusing to let them be isolated can be one of the most powerful and loving gifts you can give someone in this situation.

(Incidentally, if your friend tells you about an experi-ence that sounds to you like it was sexual assault, but they're not calling it that, you're going to want to take a very similar approach. You should never tell someone they're wrong about how they identify their experiences. But you can express your concern, ask them how they're feeling about it, connect them with resources in case they decide they want them, and tell them that if it had happened to you, you would have called it sexual assault.)

What if, instead, it's your friend who seems to be doing the *abusing*? Your approach should be similar. Don't tell them what they should or shouldn't do. Tell them what you've observed that troubles you, and why, and ask them what they think of the behaviors you're reflecting back to them. If they're troubled, too, you have an opening to help them get help. (Check out www.wyrrw.com/forabusers for some great places to start.) But if they don't see what you see, there's little you can do. Trying to force them to change behaviors they don't want to change isn't going to help anyone. It may, in fact, put the person they're hurting at greater risk—some abusers will take it out on their victims if they're challenged or confronted by a third party. So tread lightly. If you try to go in like an avenging hero, you may have the opposite effect from the one you intend.

There is one way your approach may differ: You're under no obligation to stay friends with someone who's abusing their partner. That's a personal decision. Maybe you feel you can do more good by sticking around, or maybe the friendship is old and deep and hard to give up. But if you don't want to stand by this person, that doesn't make you a bad friend. It makes you a person with boundaries.

Dive In: Write about a time you were worried about a friend's relationship. That time could be now, or use any example from the past. What was it that had you concerned? What did you do about that concern? How did the situation turn out? How would you handle it differently if you had it to do over?

If the situation is in the present tense, use the role-playing options from chapter 7 to role-play a conversation with the friend that you're worried about, using the

> guidelines outlined above. If the situation is in the past,
> role-play a different ending—give yourself a chance to try
> an approach that you wish you'd thought of then.

SLUT-SHAMING AND PRUDE-POLICING

One of the most common ways friends and family may do harm
to each other around sexuality is through slut-shaming and
prude-policing. As we explored in chapter 2, "slut-shaming" is
an umbrella term for all kinds of language and behaviors that
are intended to make women and girls feel bad about being
sexual. Of course, everyone has a slightly different definition of
the word "slut," but it hardly matters what the shamer's definition of "slut" is, because none of the related behaviors are any
of their business.

It's not for any of us to decide the moral value of another
person based on anything they may be doing in the realm of
consensual sexuality.

Why does this matter so much? Because slut-shaming does
real damage. It makes women mistrust other women. It can
make us less likely to be honest with ourselves or others about
what we want or what we're doing sexually, and that kind of
isolation can be dangerous, especially if we're in an abusive situation but don't let anyone know we need help, or if it means
we wind up without critical resources for preventing pregnancy
and STDs.

Slut-shaming also hurts women when we *do* speak up for
ourselves. Beyond the real hurt that comes from being ostra-
cized by their friends or community, women who are considered

"slutty" can find their legal rights in jeopardy. (Like the woman who was at a bar where the exploitative Girls Gone Wild video series was filming, when someone nonconsensually pulled up her shirt for the camera. When the footage turned up in one of the videos for sale, she sued, but the court ruled against her, basically saying that a single woman at a bar where Girls Gone Wild was filming should expect whatever she gets.[1] In other words: A good girl wouldn't have been there, so that's what you get for being bad.) As we discussed in chapter 2, when rape survivors press charges, we're also routinely accused of being sluts and thus "asking for it," which inspires justice systems to ignore rape allegations, which in turn allows rapists to go free and rape more women.

Slut-shaming also plays into the myth that a woman's value is tied up in what we do or don't do with our bodies. Which brings me to slut-shaming's sister: prude-policing. As much as sluts are set up for suffering in our culture, women who are perceived as having no (or not much) sexual experience can also be subjected to abuse, depending on our age or what kinds of communities we're part of. This can have an equally damaging effect, pushing women to do things sexually that we don't want to do, just to silence our critics. That often results in unsafe sexual practices and further alienation from our own actual desires (or lack thereof)—we've already explored the damaging cycle that occurs when we override our own boundaries, and that can result from prude-policing, too.

Slut-shaming and prude-policing often collide into one giant mixed message about how women should be sexual, as Zeinab discovered.

Growing up, I definitely internalized a lot of what I was taught, especially by the Catholic Church. Wanting to remain a virgin was something that was very very important to me. And there were a lot of things that if I did them, I worried they might make me less attractive to a potential husband. Then I got older, and I realized that I actually really wanted to have sex, and I didn't know how to go about doing that, so I would talk to people about it, and I had this one male friend who would tell me, "Just grab any guy! He'll be ready to go!" It felt like I was receiving a mixed message, in that it's good not to be a "slut" or a "whore," but every man will be willing to get down, and that will decrease my stock in the world.

What matters most here is that you don't let anyone define your value as a person by what you do or don't do sexually, and that you don't place those judgments on other people, either. It can be tempting. Defining ourselves as "not like" other women makes us think we won't have to suffer the consequences we may see them suffering. We may think that if we're not "slutty," we'll be safe from rape or STDs or pregnancy. Or that if we're not a "prude," we'll be popular and loved and have all the attention we need. As you know by now, the truth is much more complicated than that. Judging others for their sexual choices creates mistrust and isolation among women, when we could be helping each other out instead.

If this dynamic is playing out among your friends or family, you may need to be the first one to speak out against it. If you're not sure how to broach the subject, review the strategies for speaking up that we went over in chapter 7, and use your personal communication strength, whether that's humor, bluntness, telling on yourself, or something else.

It's hard to say what you'll find: Some people may resist, not wanting to believe they're engaging in anything but "harmless gossip." Others may be relieved that someone said something, as they were also feeling uncomfortable but didn't know what to do about it. Whatever the case, you'll at least be sending yourself the message that judgment has no place in your sexuality.

Dive In: With your nondominant hand, write out the nasty voices telling you you're a slut or a prude or any other term that pins your self-worth to your sexuality. These may be things people have explicitly said to you, or just messages you've absorbed from the culture at large. Let 'er rip—write all the most shocking or hurtful things you've ever heard said about you or believed about yourself. When you're done, take a deep breath and read back what you've written. Then, with your dominant hand, respond to the vitriol. Take all the time you need. Tell those voices exactly why they're wrong, and how they've made you feel in the past, and how you feel now, and then tell them you're not going to listen anymore. You're not going to let them hurt you anymore.

SETTING BOUNDARIES

Your friends and family may be flawlessly supportive about your sexuality. If so, congrats—you're really lucky. Because odds are, your friends and family were also raised in a toxic sexual culture and have developed any number of responses to it, some of which may be in direct opposition to what you believe or how you want to live. They may judge you or lecture you—they may even believe they're doing it for your own good. Some of them, while meaning well, may violate your physical boundaries with unwelcome hugs, uncomfortable kisses, and other intrusions. And, sadly, some of them may not mean well and may instead be emotionally or physically abusive, or may have abused you in the past.

You already have the skills you need to set boundaries with your friends and family. You learned boundary-setting skills in chapter 4, and they apply here as well. What you may not have is the belief that it's okay to tell your loved ones to stop harming you.

Reread your definition of love that you wrote in chapter 5, and then think about that sentence for a moment. Using your definition of love, would someone who loves you want to harm you? That's ultimately for you to decide, but my opinion on the matter is clear: no. Of course we all accidentally hurt each other sometimes, no matter how much we love each other. But if "love" is a verb, as I believe it is, then someone who really loves you will want to know that they've hurt you, so they can make it up to you and avoid it in the future, if at all possible.

What I'm proposing here is that a version of the Nice Person Test is the best way to approach your friends and family, too.

If someone who's supposed to love you is hurting you, either directly hurting your feelings or violating your physical boundaries, or inadvertently hurting you by pushing the Terrible Trio on you, put yourself in their shoes and ask yourself: If I was doing this to someone I love, would I want to know about it? I'm guessing you would. So act as though that's true in this case as well. Tell them, respectfully, clearly, and lovingly, what bothers you about their behavior. Then pay attention to what you can learn from their response.

This is tricky stuff emotionally. I don't mean to suggest that it's easy. I don't even mean to suggest that if your mother reacts badly when you try to talk with her about the sex shame she's been pushing on you that she doesn't love you. Obviously, it's more complicated than that. Your mother has lived her whole life with a set of beliefs, and she may well think you're in danger if you're not adhering to them. It might be very unsettling to hear that her critiques of your wardrobe, which, in her eyes, are meant to keep you out of danger, are something that you experience as harming. So have compassion. Try to see her intentions in the context of what you know of her sexual values, which may be very different from yours. In fact, if you suspect that the issue really lies in your incompatible sexual values (maybe your mother believes that only girls with low self-esteem have sex before marriage, or that going out late and drinking is going to "get you" raped), it could be most productive to try to talk about those values, and not just about the behaviors that stem from them.

"My mother's advice about when to have sex was always 'when you feel ready for it and are in a good, loving relationship,'" recalls Avory.

For a long time, I thought this was great advice because it was a sensible alternative to the "waiting for marriage" thing, and seemed to be promoting healthy behaviors— love is good, right? It wasn't until many years later that I realized this taught me that monogamy is the only option, that love is the only thing you need for sex to be great, and that there is some sort of black-line difference between a romantic relationship and a great, trusting friendship. Over time, I started to see that her well-meaning advice was steeped in one particular idea of how romantic relationships are supposed to work, and learned that for me, sex depends principally on trust and ability to comfortably communicate with someone— whether friend or romantic partner, and no matter how many relationships I have at the time.

Keep in mind that no one changes their values overnight, and lots of people won't change them at all, no matter what you say. Also remember that you may not be perfect at talking about this, either. These conversations can get emotional and heated, even if everyone has the best of intentions.

Ultimately, you've got three basic choices for dealing with people in your life who don't support your sexual health:

1. **Engage.** If the relationship is important to you, and if it seems like the person you're dealing with also cares about the relationship and wants to find a way not to hurt you, I really encourage you to try to talk it through. This can take a while. You might even want to get a neutral third party involved to

help. When I came out as queer to my parents, it got messy really fast. I never doubted that they loved me, but they really struggled to support and accept me the way I needed them to. There were tears. There were fights. Some of them were ugly. But we all hung in and kept trying to get to a better place with each other, and eventually, over the course of a few years, we really did. It was hard work for all of us, but it was worth it. We have a better, more honest relationship now than we did before. That doesn't happen for everyone, but it's possible for many.

2. **Agree to disagree.** If things get too difficult, it may be useful to back off the conversation for a while, or altogether. If you can both manage it, try agreeing to not talk about the sticky issue. This works best with an explicit conversation in which you agree on exactly what types of conversations or comments are off-limits. (So, you might say to your roommate, "You don't comment on what I'm wearing, and I won't tell you about what I do when I go out.") You can also decide if this is a permanent arrangement or if you want to try it for a period of time and then reopen the conversation once you've both had time to think and cool down. Of course, the tricky part is sticking to it.

3. **Disengage from the relationship.** This may mean cutting the person off altogether, or just keeping your distance and engaging in polite conversation only when socially required to. If a family member has been emotionally or physically abusive to you, especially if they refuse any accountability for their actions, this can sometimes be your best option. If

you want to leave the door open for the possibility of future reconciliation, you can do this with
conditions ("I'm not speaking with you until you
acknowledge and apologize for the way you treated
me"), or you can do it unconditionally. The older
and/or more important the relationship is between
you, the harder this can be to do. But you'll know
it when it's time to cross this bridge. Trust your
instincts. If you're dealing with physical or emotional abuse, consider this option if you think the
person who's harming you doesn't care that you're
getting hurt and is uninterested in stopping or negotiating. Also consider it if just being near this person
is too painful for you, even if you think their intentions toward you are benign.

Of course, none of our relationships exist in a vacuum, and
other people who know you both may try to get involved. This
can be either helpful or hard, depending on so many things.
It may be that cutting one person out of your life means that
other people cut you off. But it may also be that, say, opening a
conversation about slut-shaming with one of your friends leads
other friends to engage in that same useful conversation. You're
going to have to deal with the fallout in each of your relationships as it arises.

Dive In: Make a list of three to five family
members or friends whose attitudes toward sexuality
negatively impact you. Write down how they behave,
what they believe or say that hurts you, and how you wish

it could be different. Be as specific as you can. Now, circle the name of the person who seems most likely to be open to finding out how they're impacting you. Using the role-playing options from chapter 7, role-play a conversation with the person about what's bothering you—their false assumptions about your sexuality, the way their behavior toward other women affects you, their controlling behavior—whatever it is. But before you start, review the strategies in chapter 7 for helping yourself initiate a difficult conversation, and think about what outcome would be satisfying to you and what outcomes would be acceptable. Write those down, too. Remember to use the Nice Person Test: Tell them about it the way you'd want to hear about it if you were hurting them but didn't know you were. Let them know you value the relationship and you trust their intentions, which is why this conversation is important. Use a shit sandwich if it helps.

HOW TO TALK TO KIDS

There may be any number of situations where you have the responsibility to talk to children about sex. I'm not going to tell you what to say to them—there are just too many factors. How old is the child in question? What's your relationship to them? If you're not their parent or guardian, do you share their parent/guardian's values about sex, and if not, is it okay with the Head Grownup in charge of this child for you to share your own values? And if it isn't, what are the circumstances when it's worth doing anyhow?

So many questions, a lot of which you're going to ultimately have to answer for yourself. But I can share a few guidelines I like to follow.

- Be honest. If a child asks you a question about sex, and you can't answer it because they're just not old enough to understand, or because you're not sure it's your place to do so, tell them straight up. Don't lie. Kids can smell lies from a mile away. So if you lie to them about sex, they're going to get (a) false, confusing, made-up information about a really important subject, and (b) the feeling that they can't trust you.

- Teach them that their relationship with their bodies and their sexuality is the most important one. When they're young, that means that they get to say no if they don't want Grandpa to kiss them at Thanksgiving, even if that causes awkwardness with Grandpa. You may need to talk this over with Grandpa in advance if you think it's going to be an issue. So do it. Because Grandpa's hurt feelings aren't more important than a child's learning that they get final say over who does what to their body.

- Teach them that there's so much more to them than sexuality. For such a repressed culture, we spend a lot of our collective energy evaluating who's more important or powerful based on who's sexy. The best way to counteract this isn't to tell kids that sex is bad or dangerous and they should never even think about it, because this not only makes it seem more taboo (and therefore more compelling), but also does nothing to counteract the idea

that sexuality is the most important thing about
them. Instead, give them positive attention for other
things. If, for example, you've got a girl in your
life with a princess fetish, maybe role-play with her
about what it would be like to actually *rule* a kingdom, and help her learn to wield power firmly but
benevolently. Or indulge the princess stuff for an
hour, but only if she'll agree to do something with
you that's not related to princess play (like playing
soccer or completing a puzzle) for an hour after that.

- Teach them to respect other people's boundaries,
too. That means practicing enthusiastic consent
(though you don't have to call it that). Playing
rough or physical games is fine as long as everyone's
having a good time. But if somebody stops having
fun, the physical stuff has to stop immediately.

- Walk your talk. If you tell your thirteen-year-old
brother that it's not cool to tease girls about their
bodies, and then he hears you snarking to your
friends about how fat or skinny or slutty or prudish
or whatever some woman you know is, he's going
to learn that (a) you're a hypocrite and (b) it's actually totally fine (and possibly cool and grown-up) to
snark on women's bodies. Which brings me to:

- If they're confused, let them know they're not
alone. Kids tend to think that grownups have all
the answers. But while they should be able to trust
the adults in their lives to have more answers than
they themselves do, it can also be affirming for them
to know that some things are confusing, even for
grownups. Letting them know that some of the things

about sex that seem complicated or scary are actually complicated and can, in fact, involve real risk reassures them that their instincts are right and empowers them to ask more questions without feeling like they're "dumb kids." But don't forget to also . . .

- Make sure kids know that sex can be pleasurable! So much of what we tend to teach kids about sex is designed to scare them off of ever having it or even thinking about it. Of course it's important for kids to understand the real risks that come along with partnered sex, but it's also crucial that they know that people do it for a reason! If we leave pleasure out of what we teach kids about sex, we're essentially teaching them that when they do wind up feeling sexual pleasure, there's something dirty and secret about that pleasure. And we're especially teaching them that they shouldn't talk with us about it, because we either lied about it to them or don't understand. That kind of silencing from adults can lead kids to get their sexual information from each other, or from distorted sources like porn.

- Be prepared. There's no hard-and-fast rule about when a young person is ready for partnered sex. Your job is to encourage the young people in your life to find the time that works for them, and to resist pressure to "do it" because everyone else seems to be, or to "save it" just because someone else thinks they should. Instead, help young people decide for themselves using some basic guidelines: Are they comfortable talking about and acquiring the necessary supplies to practice safer sex? Are they with a partner who practices enthusiastic consent and will respect their boundaries, and are they ready to do the same for a partner? Are they genuinely excited and curious about sex? Are they emotionally strong enough to handle any fallout that might result, from heartbreak to unintended pregnancy? Heather Corinna of Scarleteen has developed a great "Sex Readiness Checklist," which you can find in her book, *S.E.X.*,[2] or at www.wyrrw .com/sexreadiness. Go over it with a young person who's thinking of dipping their toe into sexual waters—it will inspire great conversation!

Of course, by now you'll recognize that these are great sexual values to teach anyone, at any age. Because the basics don't change, whether you're eight or eighty. As Heather notes,

The biggest part of where my father did really well in teaching me about sexuality was in making clear that if I was going to be sexual with others, I needed to be able to take my own responsibility around it, which included things like seeking out my own sexual health care, safer sex, and contraception and being accountable for my own actions. He also made it clear that while those kinds of things were things I needed to do for myself (the idea being if I needed him to do them, I probably wasn't ready to be actively sexual with others), I'd always have 100 percent of his emotional support, acceptance, and advocacy as I navigated being sexual and managing my sexual life.

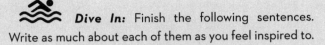 **Dive In:** Finish the following sentences. Write as much about each of them as you feel inspired to.

- The number one thing I wish someone had taught me about sex when I was growing up is:

  _____

- The best thing anyone ever taught me about sex when I was growing up was:

  _____

- The worst thing anyone ever taught me about sex when I was growing up was:

  _____

- When I was growing up, I learned the most about sex from:

  _____

- When I was growing up, what I learned about sex from watching adults was:

  _____

WINGWOMEN AND OTHER GREAT BIRDS

At the end of a chapter about the challenges of dealing with friends and family about sex, it's important to remember that the people closest to you can also be your closest allies as you go after what you really really want. Do you feel shy about flirting with people or asking them out? It all goes so much more easily if you've got a good wingwoman by your side, egging you on and helping you strategize. (Plus, even if you get rejected, you're still having a memorable experience with your friend.)

Need help learning how to trust your intuition? A trusted confidant can be an essential sounding board as you sort out generalized fears from useful instincts.

Reluctant to take a self-defense class by yourself? Go with a friend, and make a bonding experience out of it.

Trying to build up your sexual communication skills? You already know how helpful a close pal can be when you need to role-play a difficult conversation. And, of course, good friends and family are there to help you through when you suffer heartbreak, dish the details of your hot encounters, cheer you on as you steel yourself to make a tough relationship decision, and toast your joy when you find a partner that exceeds your dreams.

At one point, when I was trying to come to an understanding with my body and the fact that people did, in fact, want it, I decided to go to a club for BBWs (big beautiful women) and FAs (fat admirers). I'd put it off for ages because I didn't have a single local friend who was fat and I have a lot of anxiety issues around new places and people. So a friend of mine offered to go with me. All 105 pounds of her! The club was terrible but we had an awesome time regardless. And it was a great feeling knowing that she was willing to go outside of her comfort zone to keep me company and help me experience new things. {Heidi}

Dive In: If you didn't already do this in chapter 2 (or if you want to do it again for someone else), write a letter to a friend or family member telling them how much you value them and what it is they do that makes a difference in your life, and thanking them for supporting your pursuit of healthy sexuality.

Go Deeper:

1. Get out your timeline and add five instances in which a friend or family member impacted your sexual life. Their influence may have been helpful, damaging, or too complex to categorize. Now pick one of those instances, and spend ten minutes writing about it. Who was it, and what was your relationship like at the time? What did they do that impacted you? What did it teach you? How, if at all, has it changed your relationship with your sexuality? Do you think this person knows what an impact they had on you? Do you think they would have the same impact on you if they did a similar thing today?

2. Take a wingwoman field trip! Find a friend who supports your sexual values and go out for a night of fun together. If one or both of you is looking for a partner, try your hand at flirting (or more!)—tell each other what kind of person and experience you're looking for, and take turns scouting the talent for each other, coordinating flirtation strategies, and generally egging each other on. Don't

focus on whether or not you "get lucky" with a sex partner or not—just enjoy being lucky enough to have a great wingwoman.

If you're both partnered off, spend the night telling stories of your sexploits, confiding about struggles you might be having in the sack, or confessing fantasies you've yet to fulfill. Again, the point isn't to have the wildest story or to solve anybody's problems—just appreciate having a confidant with whom you can talk about your sexual secrets.

3. Ever read advice columns? Sure you do! They're addictive, right? They're popular for a couple of reasons: First, we can look for situations like our own. If we find them, we not only feel validated but may also be able to apply the advice given and see how we like it. Second, it's a fun challenge to read the question and, before reading the answer, try to figure out what advice we would give in response, then see how close we came, or see how our advice differs.

    So write your own! This might be a good way to work through some of the issues you see in your relationships with your friends and family. Put yourself in their shoes for a few minutes. What letter might they write to an advice column, and what might the wise columnist advise in return? You might also try writing up and answering some of your own current dilemmas. It can be good to summarize the heart of the issue quickly, to read the letter like someone else wrote it, and to respond in another persona. It helps give you perspective on the issue. Another way you can use this exercise is to actually do it with one or more of your friends and family members. You can each write a letter, about a real or fictional situation, past or present, then hand them around for replies (anonymously, if that feels better). As you share the letters and responses at the end of the exercise, it's a good segue into discussing sex and sexual issues with the people in your life. And since the letters are anonymous or even fictional, no one feels judged.

4. Wish a particular man in your life could better understand the way he influences your sexuality? Whether it's a family member, a lover, or a friend, ask him to read and complete the bonus chapter, Just For Men, which you can find at www.wyrrw.com/justformen, and then sit down and talk it over afterward.

CHAPTER 11

TO INFINITY AND BEYOND

WELCOME TO CHAPTER 11! IN U.S. BANKRUPTCY LAW, "chapter 11" refers to the part of the bankruptcy process in which the business or individual can begin to reorganize and rebuild. While we've been reorganizing in every chapter, it seems particularly appropriate in this last one. As you leave behind old and bankrupt ideas about sexuality in favor of what you really really want, it can feel unstable and chaotic. In this chapter we'll try to firm up the ground beneath you so that you can jump off from here to wherever you want to go next.

Let's start by revisiting where you were in chapter 1 and seeing what's changed and what hasn't. Remember this quiz? Without peeking at your answers from when you took it the first time, take it again now:

1. I know how to stay safe while expressing my sexuality.

   Strongly Disagree ① ② ③ ④ ⑤ ⑥ ⑦ ⑧ ⑨ ⑩ *Strongly Agree*

2. I'm afraid of what others would think/say/do if they knew how I feel about sex.

Strongly Disagree ① ② ③ ④ ⑤ ⑥ ⑦ ⑧ ⑨ ⑩ *Strongly Agree*

3. I can tell when sexual activity is making me uncomfortable.

Strongly Disagree ① ② ③ ④ ⑤ ⑥ ⑦ ⑧ ⑨ ⑩ *Strongly Agree*

4. I can tell when sexual activity is giving me pleasure.

Strongly Disagree ① ② ③ ④ ⑤ ⑥ ⑦ ⑧ ⑨ ⑩ *Strongly Agree*

5. I feel comfortable telling a potential sexual partner that something they're doing is making me uncomfortable.

Strongly Disagree ① ② ③ ④ ⑤ ⑥ ⑦ ⑧ ⑨ ⑩ *Strongly Agree*

6. I feel comfortable telling a potential sexual partner what to do in order to give me pleasure.

Strongly Disagree ① ② ③ ④ ⑤ ⑥ ⑦ ⑧ ⑨ ⑩ *Strongly Agree*

7. My sexual values make sense to me.

Strongly Disagree ① ② ③ ④ ⑤ ⑥ ⑦ ⑧ ⑨ ⑩ *Strongly Agree*

8. I often do sexual things or have sexual feelings that make me feel confused or bad.

Strongly Disagree ① ② ③ ④ ⑤ ⑥ ⑦ ⑧ ⑨ ⑩ *Strongly Agree*

9. My sexual partner(s), if I have them, share my values about sex.

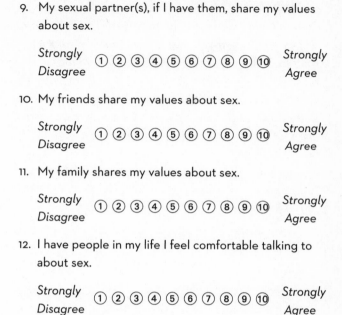

Strongly Disagree ① ② ③ ④ ⑤ ⑥ ⑦ ⑧ ⑨ ⑩ *Strongly Agree*

10. My friends share my values about sex.

Strongly Disagree ① ② ③ ④ ⑤ ⑥ ⑦ ⑧ ⑨ ⑩ *Strongly Agree*

11. My family shares my values about sex.

Strongly Disagree ① ② ③ ④ ⑤ ⑥ ⑦ ⑧ ⑨ ⑩ *Strongly Agree*

12. I have people in my life I feel comfortable talking to about sex.

Strongly Disagree ① ② ③ ④ ⑤ ⑥ ⑦ ⑧ ⑨ ⑩ *Strongly Agree*

How'd you do? Specifically, ask yourself if those answers are what you'd like them to be. If some of them aren't, go back and circle them. We'll talk about them in a minute. But first, find your answers now from when you took this quiz in chapter 1. Put a star next to every answer that's changed. Then go back and take out the commitment you made to yourself at the beginning of the book. Reread it, and think about it. Did you live up to it? Did you accomplish what you set out to do? Or at least some of it? Whatever the answer, take a moment now to appreciate all the hard work you've put into this process, and where it's led you.

Here's what Heidi had to say after completing the process:

*The main thing that I'm better at is actually sitting down
and figuring out what I want in a partner and what I
want from sex, instead of living with some vague [sense
of] Oh, I'll know it when I find it and then having no clue
what I'm actually looking for. And also just remembering
that I'm not an abandoned puppy waiting to be adopted,
and that I'm allowed to do the choosing. I've actually
had the STD talk with a couple of people, and I've can-
celed a couple of things because I wasn't sure I felt comfortable with them. I don't want to be doing things with
regret anymore.*

Dive In: Write yourself a thank-you note. Tell
yourself how much you appreciate the effort you put into
working through this book. Make sure to remind yourself why it matters that you did this work. Also be sure
to acknowledge what parts you've done particularly well,
what the hardest parts were, if there were parts where
you felt like quitting (or did quit for a while) and how
you overcame those obstacles, and what a difference it's
going to make in your life going forward. Don't be stingy
with the praise! Flatter yourself wildly.

TO BOLDLY GO

Of course, no matter how far you've come since chapter 1, you
may still have a few issues with sexuality. For most of us, sort-

ing out our relationship with our own sexuality is a lifelong journey.

Just because you've finished the book, don't feel that you have to be finished with exploring the ideas and questions we've grappled with here. Consider those answers you just circled above. They're not failures—they're signs telling you where you may want to focus your future attention. You don't have to do it all right now. Let the things you've learned so far about yourself settle in. Think about something else for a while. Then, when you feel ready, ask yourself if there are exercises in this book that address unresolved issues that you want to go deeper with. Go back and get into it. Are there exercises you wish you'd had time to do the first time but wound up skipping? Go back and try them out. Are there sections that make sense to you, but you're having trouble really internalizing them? Do them again. Are there people you wish you could have all of these conversations with? Why not drop them a line and ask them to do the book with you, starting again from chapter 1?

In other words, think of this book as a basic road map. You probably haven't gone down all of its routes yet. There may be some you'd really like to double back to and explore, and there may be some you have no interest in checking out. Some streets that you've now driven down once are going to be places you want to make part of your regular travels, and some of them may be excursions you're glad you went on but don't need to do again. And, of course, there are plenty of places not on the map of this book at all. I've pointed to some of them—the resources throughout the book where you can learn more about a wide variety of topics we had time to go into only briefly in these pages. And every one of those resources will lead you to other new places as well.

The most important thing is to feed the exploratory spirit that led you to pick up this book in the first place. Your curiosity about what's possible for your sexuality and your understanding that what people and institutions are telling you is not always the whole story (and sometimes not even the truth) are wonderful guides. Follow them, using the tools you've learned along the way:

Risk assessment

Keep in mind that there's no way to avoid risk altogether; your job is to cut through blame, shame, and fear by using reliable information to answer the following questions: How big is the risk (to you and others, emotionally and physically) in pursuing sexual things you may want to do? Are there ways you can reduce those risks, and how great might the reward be, despite the risk? How likely are the good and bad outcomes to happen? Once you have your answers in hand, you can make a decision that makes sense to you.

Intuition

Remember: Intuition is specific. It says things like, *This person seems nice, but I don't think he's trustworthy.* Generalized fear is the opposite of intuition: It says things like, *Don't trust anybody, no matter how nice they seem.* Turn down the volume on your generalized fears and amplify your intuition, and you'll be both safer and happier.

Emotional connection

Your feelings—even the uncomfortable ones—are important. They're telling you something. Treat them like clues. They may not contain answers all by themselves, but they're a crucial part of the puzzle when it comes to figuring out what you want or need. Make room for them. Make friends with them. Because even if they feel awful in the moment, when it comes to feelings, the only way out is through.

Direct communication

As awkward as it can feel to blurt out what you need to say, you can't expect people to be mind readers. Whether you're expressing a desire or setting a boundary, you can take control of your body and your sexuality only if you're willing to talk about them. Use the tools and tricks in chapter 7 to help you get the words out.

The Golden Rule

It's a classic for a reason: If you do unto others as you would have them do unto you (especially if you believe you deserve loving, respectful treatment, which you do!), you'll probably be a good friend, family member, and lover, even while you're pursuing what you really really want. (It's no accident that direct communication + the Golden Rule = the Nice Person Test.)

Please also remember that many of the things you've discovered in this book are new. You've tried on new ways of seeing yourself, your partners, your friends and family, and the world. You've experimented with new ways of behaving, new ways of talking with people, new ways of relating to your own desires, needs, and boundaries. Probably, many of these new approaches still feel, well, new. Don't get me wrong: New can be great! It can be exciting, exhilarating, liberating, energizing! But it can also feel unfamiliar. Inauthentic. Uncomfortable. Awkward. Artificial.

One of the greatest gifts you can give yourself right now is time. Time to try on these new approaches long enough to see if they begin to feel more comfortable and natural. Don't forget— you've been working on this book for a few months, maybe. But you've had the old behaviors, the ones you may now be trying to change, for many years. It makes a lot of sense that they might feel more comfortable. But "comfortable" doesn't mean those behaviors and beliefs are working well for you. If they were, you probably would never have picked up this book in the first place.

One of my first girlfriends taught me this valuable framework for thinking about learning new ways of being: You start off in *unconscious incompetence*. That is, you're not being effective on your own behalf, and you're not even aware of what you're doing wrong. As you begin to learn, you shift into *conscious incompetence*. This can be the most uncomfortable stage of learning new ways of being. You're aware that you're doing things that aren't good for you, but you can't seem to stop doing them, out of force of habit, fear of change, etc. But don't give up! Because the next stage is *conscious competence*. That's when, if you focus on it deliberately, you can do things a new and healthier way. This is the part where it feels awkward and artificial, even though you're acting in a way that you know is better for you. And if you do that for long enough, you'll eventually find your way into *unconscious competence*—that fantastic sweet spot where the things that feed your soul feel so natural that you do them without even thinking about them.

So hang in there with the weird, awkward feelings. And give yourself permission to be imperfect. It would be surprising if you didn't sometimes revert to old behaviors or beliefs that you've tried to shed over the course of this book. Growth isn't linear. You don't move from one step to another in that four-step learning curve I just outlined without ever slipping back and forth a little. We learn things, and then we backslide a little and we have to learn them again in a new way. Don't give up if you catch yourself acting or thinking in a way that's not compatible with what you really really want. Just notice it, see if there's anything to learn from it, and let it go. There's always a new opportunity to move from conscious incompetence to conscious competence again the next time around.

Here's Mieko's plan going forward:

I've gotten better at trusting my intuition more, especially around my male friends. I'm a lot calmer around them now, because I'm more confident in my boundaries with myself. But I'm still not so confident with strangers. So one of the ways I'm going to deal with that is that I'm going to take a self-defense class. That way I can be confident walking down the street and knowing that not only does nobody have the right to come up to me and touch me without my permission, but if somebody tries it, I can do

WHAT YOU REALLY REALLY WANT

something about it. That's definitely the next step for me. I also want to invest more in doing things that give me pleasure. I might buy myself a new sex toy or something!

All of the challenges you may still face are a great reason to keep doing your weekly body love and daily writing, even though you're "officially" done with this process. (Or hey, if you weren't keeping up with them while you worked on the book, there's no time like the present to start.) There's never a bad reason to focus on giving yourself physical pleasure or carving out ten minutes a day to get in tune with your thoughts by spilling them onto a page. But now is an especially good time to keep up these practices—this can be a delicate transitional moment, and anything that helps you stay grounded and focused on what you really really want will be a real asset. So don't stop now, and if you need to, start again: Love your body every week, and do a little private freewriting every day. It's a good way to be your own best friend.

Dive In: Make a new commitment to yourself to make the lessons you've learned through this process last. Start by writing down what you've learned about yourself, your sexuality, and the world you're living in. Write down everything you can think of. Now, make a list of anything you still feel uncertain or challenged about— anything you still want or need to figure out. You don't have to do it all now! Just list everything you can think of.

Now, just as you did in chapter 1, send yourself a message. Tell yourself what you plan to do now to make sure the lessons you've learned aren't lost, and what you plan to do to support yourself on your ongoing journey. Don't forget to send your future self a message about why continuing this work is important, what you've already gotten out of it, what you want to get out of it in the future, and what you want your future self to remember when things start to feel hard. Say whatever you want, but also be sure to include the following sentences: "I, [your name], am making a promise to myself: I won't give up on seeking out what I really really want. Because I matter to myself. My desires matter, my pleasure matters, and my safety matters. This process is a gift to myself, and I promise to keep accepting it."

GROW TOGETHER

Of course, if you have to give yourself some leeway to settle into the new you, that means your friends and family will almost certainly need some as well. Almost nobody likes change, especially in the ones we love. So if you're doing things differently as a result of this book (perhaps you're being more direct about what you want and don't want, or you're dressing differently, or your desires themselves have changed) and you experience some blowback from the people around you, try to be patient. That doesn't mean you have to put up with people treating you badly. But keep in mind that people still living in the throes of shame, blame, and fear are likely to feel, at some level, like you're challenging their worldview if they see you rejecting the Terrible Trio. So set boundaries with them if you need to. If it feels like they'd be open to it, sit them down and explain to them why you're changing and how their response is affecting you. Definitely don't let them talk you out of pursuing a happier, healthier sexuality just because it makes them uncomfortable. But if they seem to be trying to understand, have compassion for them, too. It may even be useful to share this book with them—if they're women, they may have a lot to learn from it. And if they're men, there's a special section at www.wyrrw .com/justformen that will help them understand how they can be more supportive of you.

These changes may be especially challenging if you have one or more ongoing sexual partners. Don't get me wrong: They may also be awesome. You may already have found that they've improved your sexual satisfaction and strengthened your relationship in general. But if you change the way you go about your sexual relationships, you're also changing the way your partner's sexual relationship works. And while you chose this process you're both now engaged in, they may not have.

It may be that working through this book has helped you to see your partner in a different light. Perhaps you've discovered that they're not very interested in your desires or your boundaries. That's difficult information to learn about anyone, let alone someone you're already intimate with. That kind of disregard is not something you need to put up with. On the other hand, you may be pleasantly surprised to discover how well your partner responds to your developing sense of your sexuality. Their responses to your new ways of behaving and communicating may increase the trust between you, strengthening the ties you already have.

But if their response falls somewhere in between—if they're supportive of the reasons you're changing but having trouble adjusting to it in practice—try to cut them a little slack for a while. As we discussed in chapter 9, make sure you're compromising *with them*, as opposed to compromising *yourself*. But if you can find ways to make room for them to work through their discomfort without sacrificing too much of yourself, you could be doing both of you a favor, allowing the relationship to grow to meet both of your needs.

That's exactly what Prerna and her boyfriend are doing. "Because this is my first serious relationship after being sexually assaulted, how I handled the sexual aspects of it was an entirely new territory that I didn't expect," she says.

My boyfriend was so understanding and kind and in my head I assumed everything would be happily wonderful in bed, too, and I led him to believe that. But I quickly came to realize that things weren't as fine as I'd thought they would be. I ended up in tears every time we had sex, and not the good kind! When I first tried to talk about it with him, he was upset because he didn't want to be hurting me in any way, but also because he thought I was putting the kibosh on sex. And at first that was exactly what I did. I didn't know how to deal with my feelings, so preventing them from coming up by not having sex in the first place seemed like a good idea. He was patient with me, but it quickly became clear that it wasn't working for either of us. Eventually we decided to try things again, but slowly and with lots of pauses to make sure we were both feeling good and content with what we were doing. That was so much better! There are still kinks we're ironing out, but now that we're on the same page we're both less afraid to speak up about what works and what doesn't.

As for finding new partners, keep in mind what we talked about in the introduction: This book isn't designed to make it easier for you to find sexual partners. What it will do is make it easier to distinguish partners who'll be good for you from ones who won't, and to make your experience better when you do find a good partner. The sad reality is that since we've all been raised in a dysfunctional sexual culture, many of your potential partners may have unrealistic and sometimes damaging ideas about women and sex. (This may be more likely if your potential partners are male, but it's possible no matter what gender your partners are.) As you get clearer about what you really really want and what you really really don't, it can result in a smaller pool of people to pick from. That sucks, plain and simple. But it also means that when you do get with someone, you're far more likely to have a healthy, satisfying experience, whether it's a flirtation, a one-night stand, or a long-term partnership.

Whether you've already got a partner or are still on the lookout, you're ultimately going to have to decide how much you're willing to "educate" them, versus how much you want them to already understand and care about your sexual priorities. If you're with someone who believes women who go out wearing a short skirt are "asking to be raped," is that a deal breaker for you, or a teachable moment? If your partner thinks it's unsexy to talk openly about sex, is that the beginning of an important conversation for the two of you, or the end of the road? You're totally justified in feeling like it's not your job to teach your partners how to not be sexist, nor is it your responsibility to be their personal sex educator. If you choose the zero-tolerance route, you may have a harder time finding folks who meet your standards, but you'll have less work to do in your relationships when you do have them. On the other hand, if you're willing to take on "fixer-uppers" who are curious and well-meaning but need you to help out with some enlightenment, you'll find more willing candidates, but you'll be putting in more effort and taking a bigger gamble. There's no right answer. The right balance is up to you.

Dive In: Complete the following sentences. Feel free to write as much or as little as you like about each:

- The person who's been the most supportive to me throughout this process is:

  _____

- The person who seems most challenged by the ways I'm changing is:

  _____

- I wish I could make _____ understand that:

  _____

- I've been most surprised by how _____ reacted to:

  _____

- The person I most need to talk with more about all of this is _____. I really want us to talk about:

  _____

PAY IT FORWARD

Now that you've got a stronger grip on how to know what you really really want (and how to go after it), you may stop and think to yourself, *Why does this have to be so hard?* It's not fair that the way our culture is structured makes it difficult for us to just be ourselves. If that makes you feel angry, frustrated, or sad, you're not alone. And while there's nothing you can do to change the past, there's plenty you can do to change the future, so that the generation of women growing up after you get a lot less of the Terrible Trio, and a lot more of what they really really want, from the outset.

The media's a great place to start. Pay attention to the types of media you're consuming. Video games, music, movies, TV, books, even porn—they exist because you give them money to exist. So think about the kinds of messages they're sending you and everyone else, and vote with your dollars. In other words: Give your money to media that portrays the kind of world you want to live in, and stiff the rest. Not only will you wind up consuming media that supports your values—an awesome goal in and of itself—but you'll also have a role in creating a world where more of that media exists for other people to find.

(Of course, you can indulge in "guilty pleasures" sometimes. We all have guilty media pleasures. But be aware when you're doing it, and, when possible, do it in ways that don't give money to people perpetrating shame, blame, and fear.)

Another place you may want to get involved is in shaping the way sex education is taught in schools. Think back to your own sex ed class: How helpful was it? Did you learn that sex was something good girls Just Don't Do until marriage, and that was that? Or did you learn that if you insist on having sex, you'd better be super-careful, because otherwise you'll wind up pregnant and with all sorts of nasty diseases? Those are the two dominant models in the United States right now, and they're both missing something crucial: pleasure. As we discussed in chapter 10, if you talk to kids about sex and don't mention pleasure, it creates suspicion, shame, silence, and secrecy. It certainly doesn't make you seem credible: By the time kids are exposed to sex ed in school, even if they're not having sex, they have a sense that it might feel pretty great when they do. But leaving pleasure out of sex education does something even worse: It tells women that our satisfaction is an afterthought.

Think about it: In "prevention-based" sex education, the kind about condoms and preventing diseases and pregnancy, the act that's focused on is penis-in-vagina intercourse. Even if pleasure isn't mentioned, this teaches boys about the primary way to get sexual pleasure—through stimulation of the penis. But most women don't reach orgasm from vaginal stimulation alone. Nearly two-thirds of all women require stimulation of the clitoris in order to get off.

And the clitoris is an amazing organ! It's the only organ in the human body, male or female, that has pleasure as its sole purpose. Awesome, right? But you'll never learn about it in "harm reduction" sex ed classes, because you don't have to talk about the clitoris in order to teach people to prevent STDs and pregnancy. I don't know about you, but in my high school, the clitoris wasn't even on the anatomy drawing. No wonder so many of us grow up thinking sex is something women do for men's pleasure.[1]

If you want the next generation to grow up with a healthier, more well-rounded vision of sexuality, find out what your local school district (or the school district of a young person you care about) is teaching in terms of sex ed. If they're not teaching a holistic, pleasure-based model, encourage them to think about it. Then ask your friends and family members who agree with you to encourage them, too.

> **Dive In:** Check out some people and organizations working to create a healthier sexual culture for all of us. Spend at least thirty minutes on one or more of the websites listed at www.wyrrw.com/sexposorgs.

STRENGTH IN NUMBERS

Did you know that if a female bonobo, a kind of ape, is being subjected to unwelcome sexual aggression by a male bonobo, she gives out a specific signal and the other females will come to her aid until the male is repelled? The bonobos are very sexually active animals, but that doesn't mean that the females have to accept sexual attention from all males at all times. And they keep it that way by having each other's backs.

Wouldn't it be fantastic if more human women did that for each other? If we not only refrained from slut-shaming, prude-policing, victim-blaming, and other ways in which we hurl the Terrible Trio at each other, but actively came to each other's defense when others tried to do the same?

It can sometimes feel scary to do. If you jump in to defend someone else, whatever nastiness was being directed their way may suddenly be targeted at you. But if we're ever going to really change the sexual culture, we have to start standing up for other women's rights to do what they really really want, not just our own.

As Shana learned, this isn't always easy, but it can be very rewarding:

I was working a restaurant opening in Miami last year, and one of the girls I worked with became the subject of the rumor/gossip mill. She had at that point slept with five or six members of the staff over a month or so period, and the "slut" and "whore" comments were flying. I found myself at one point having those same opinions, and it actually scared me how easy it was to get wrapped up in group dismissals and judgments of people's sexual choices.

I had to stop and really question why I was allowing myself to think like that. I realized that since she was ex-military as well, it was triggering all the feelings and issues I had dealt with in the military. Without doing anything, I was judged to be a slut while I was in the military. The statement has been made since WWII: Why would women want to be in the military, if not to sleep around with all those available men? Being treated like that for long periods of time is exhausting. I thought that I had worked through those feelings, but finding myself participating in sexually shaming another woman made me realize that I wasn't really as past those feelings as I thought I was.

The end of this tale, though, is that once I realized why I was having that reaction, I realized how awful and unlike me I was acting. I started defending her to those around me, and reminding people that everyone has a right to do what they want sexually. If it doesn't affect you, back off. Especially when these shaming state-ments are being made by male bartenders who are on a constant pickup quest from their post behind the bar. So, it's okay for you to take home a different girl every night, but not for her? The girl and I actually became very good friends after I moved past my issues and got to know her, instead of the image other people were por-traying of her.

You don't have to do it every time there's an opportunity—no one's perfect, and life is complicated. But if you start looking for opportunities to stand up for other women, you'll not only help out in the situation at hand, but also set an example that will make it easier for those other women to stand up for some-one else—maybe even you—the next time around.

> **Dive In:** This one's simple, but not necessar-ily easy: Make a pact with a woman you care about that you'll always have each other's backs when it comes to people's blaming, shaming, or mistreating you. Then do it.

DIFFICULT CONVERSATIONS

We've already talked about how to have difficult conversations with your loved ones about your sexual values, and we've talked about reasons to have those conversations that benefit you and your partners directly. But another reason to have these heart-to-hearts is because they have the power to change the sexual culture for everyone.

Think about the modern LGBT-rights movement in the United States and elsewhere. While queer people still face many kinds of oppression, much of the progress that's been made in undoing LGBT discrimination over the past twenty years was made possible because millions of people came out to the people around them. They sat down and had the difficult conversations required to live their lives openly and free of shame, blame, and fear. These conversations didn't always go well. Many of them took years to resolve, and some people paid a very high price for them. But what they bought was a culture where most people know someone—a relative, a friend, a coworker, a neighbor, someone—who's gay, lesbian, bi, queer, or trans. And that means that there are a whole lot more people in the world who take it personally when LGBT people face discrimination, oppression, or violence.

Similarly, if you want the next generation of young women to build their sexuality in a world much freer from the Terrible Trio, one of the best things you can do is sit down with people who care about you, but who don't share your sexual values, and explain to them why you believe what you do, and why it's important to you for them to understand your point of view. As we've discussed before, it may not go well at first, or at all. But you'll get through at least some of the time. And that person you influence will also naturally influence others around them. And that ripple effect will eventually make the world a lot safer for all of us to be sexual on our own terms. Isn't that ultimately what we all really really want?

 Go Deeper:

1.   Take out your timeline and spend some time looking at it. What story does it tell about your sexual life so far? Are there pieces missing that are important to you? Fill them in now. Then think about the next five years, or ten. What story do you want your timeline to tell as you move forward in your life? Draw in some more years, and fill in at least three points in the future that you'd like to see happen. Let your imagination go wild. Anything is possible.

2.   There are countless types of journeys. Some are eventful and some less so, but even a trip to the store to buy milk can turn into an adventure. We like to read and watch stories about journeys— from *The Lord of the Rings* to *Hannah Montana*.

     This book has been something of a journey, too, and I invite you to write it like an epic adventure, with you as the hero.

     Here's a classic journey narrative:

     a.   The hero has a mission—she wants to find something precious.

     b.   She assembles all the stuff she'll need for the trip and sets out on her quest to find what she really really wants.

c. She may take some friends along for the ride, but that's optional.

d. She encounters difficulties—maybe she gets tempted down the wrong path and gets lost. Maybe she runs into a few shady characters. Maybe sometimes she falls for glittery temptations and forgets why she even set out.

e. Sometimes she is helped by people along the way. Some of these folk are mystical beings (think Yoda) who speak in riddles and don't seem that helpful at first.

f. Usually the hero has to pass some kind of test. She is tempted, but refuses. She is scared, but she forges right ahead. Sometimes she even slips a little, but at the last moment, she climbs out of her hole and marches across the finish line.

g. She comes home. She has made it. Her journey is complete.

NOTES

CHAPTER 1

YOU CAN'T GET WHAT YOU WANT TILL
YOU KNOW WHAT YOU WANT

1   See www.time.com/time/magazine/article/0,9171,1101040607-644153,00.html.

2   See www.idahopress.com/news/article_d6a73c14-1eea-11e0-9f44-001cc4c03286.html.

3   See http://kateharding.net/faq/but-dont-you-realize-fat-is-unhealthy/.

CHAPTER 2

BAD THINGS COME IN THREES:
SHAME, BLAME, AND FEAR

1   A small percentage of people are asexual, meaning they have no desire to engage in sexual activity. You can learn more about asexuality at www.asexuality.org.

2   See www.washingtoncitypaper.com/articles/1859/nice-ass.

3   See http://jezebel.com/5608138/
    what-you-were-wearing-when-you-were-sexually-harassed.

4   See http://en.wikipedia.org/wiki/
    Hate_crime_laws_in_the_United_States.

5 See www.nytimes.com/2011/03/09/us/09assault.html.

6 See http://m.theglobeandmail.com/news/national/christie-blatchford/
in-manitoba-sexual-assault-means-having-to-say-youre-sorry/
article1937678/?service=mobile.

7 See https://yesmeansyesblog.wordpress.com/2009/11/12/
meet-the-predators/.

8 pp. 113–14.

CHAPTER 3

I'M OKAY, YOU'RE OKAY

1 See www.slate.com/id/2174850/.

2 p. 123.

3 See http://consumerist.com/2007/12/walmart-junior-panties-suggest-
that-your-genitals-are-better-than-credit-cards.html.

4 See www.dailymail.co.uk/femail/article-1365461/Sex-no-half-women-
feeling-fat.html.

5 p. 117.

6 See http://shakespearessister.blogspot.com/2011/03/on-surviving-and-
sex-ed.html.

CHAPTER 4

A WOMAN'S INTUITION

1 I'm going to use "they," "their," and "them" throughout the book
to refer to a person whose gender isn't specified—like here, where the
friend you're writing to could be male, female, genderqueer, etc. The
grammar nerd in me isn't a fan, but at the moment they seem to be the
easiest gender-neutral pronouns for all people to understand.

2 See https://yesmeansyesblog.wordpress.com/2009/11/12/
meet-the-predators/.

3 See http://althouse.blogspot.com/2006/09/lets-take-closer-look-at-those-breasts.html#comments.

4 See http://web.cecs.pdx.edu/~tellner/sd/Review.html.

CHAPTER 5

WHAT'S LOVE GOT TO DO WITH IT?

1 p. 227.

2 See www.campusprogress.org/articles/moral_panic_comes_unhooked.

3 See www.cbn.com/cbnnews/healthscience/2010/march/sexually-indulgent-now-marriage-ruined-later/.

4 See www.apa.org/monitor/feb08/oxytocin.aspx.

5 See www.cdc.gov/nchs/pressroom/01news/firstmarr.htm.

CHAPTER 6

FREAKS AND GEEKS

1 Just as you do in real life, you're likely to encounter people in virtual worlds who think it's fun or normal to treat women poorly. This behavior is sometimes exacerbated by the anonymity online venues provide. If you come across this sort of ugly behavior, feel free to use it as an opportunity to practice boundary setting (remember the Nice Person Test?), or ignore it, or tell the person off in a way you never would in real life. If behavior is particularly offensive, you can also report it to the folks who run the site you're on, usually through their "help" or "contact" section.

CHAPTER 7

LET'S TALK ABOUT SEX, BABY

1 See www.thedailybeast.com/blogs-and-stories/2011-01-25/jane-mcgonigals-reality-is-broken-how-videogames-change-the-world/.

2 "Red Lights, Big Names," *CIO* (June 15, 2007): 50.

CHAPTER 8
IT'S COMPLICATED

1   FetLife is the Facebook of kink communities, but some find it cliquish and hard to navigate. It's a place to connect with like-minded people, but do proceed at your own risk.

2   From www.friendly-ware.com/wellness/images/WellnessWheel.gif.

CHAPTER 9
DO UNTO OTHERS

1   Some people who don't identify with the male/female binary use "ze" and "hir" to refer to themselves, as Enoch does. They're a new kind of gender-neutral pronoun.

CHAPTER 10
FRIENDS AND FAMILY

1   See www.stltoday.com/news/local/metro/article_30865bcc-95eb-11df-9734-00127992bc8b.html.

2   p. 127.

CHAPTER 11
TO INFINITY AND BEYOND

1   For the definitive essay on this subject, read Cara Kulwicki's "Real Sex Education" in *Yes Means Yes*.

ACKNOWLEDGMENTS

No one deserves more gratitude for their contributions to this book than the eleven volunteers who jumped into this journey with me and workshopped every chapter as I finished it. Their directly quoted words are some of the best things in this book, and their influence and inspiration have shaped every page. Prerna Abbi, Robin Colodzin, Judith Avory Faucette, Mieko Gavia, Rayshauna Gray, Rebecca Kling, Heidi Knabe, Shana Minish, Zeinab O., Enoch Riese, and Buffy Seipel, I'll never be able to fully express my gratitude to you for your honesty, bravery, humor, dedication, camaraderie, intelligence, and thoughtfulness. You gave so much more to this project than I had ever dared to hope for or even imagine.

Also essential to the making of this book was educator extraordinaire Claire Robson, who created almost all of the "Go Deeper" exercises throughout the book, as well as the timeline. Without her provocative and compassionate contributions, this road map to healthy sexuality would have outlined a much smaller world. And without her friendship and mentoring over more than a decade, I could never have written this or any book.

Thomas MacAulay Millar not only contributed the excellent section for men that can be found online at www.wyrrw.com/formen (and pulled together a fantastic group of guys to workshop it—big thanks to Daniel J. Corcoran, David Mortman, Daetan Huck, Jason Page, Oliver Lauenstein, Nick, Gabriel Pastrana, Ben Privot, and Admin Dave), but also served as a steady sounding board, talked me off several metaphorical ledges, and continues to be an invaluable comrade.

I'm blessed to have as friends some outrageously smart and dedicated people whose expertise I've relied on throughout this process. Much love and gratitude are owed to: Heather Corinna, for being this book's literal godmother, a generous host, and an international treasure who's dedicated her life to providing countless thousands (possibly millions) of people with the support and straightforward information they need to live lives full of safety and pleasure. Mylène St. Pierre, for sharing with me the wisdom of her many years as a whip-smart sex educator, and for her big-ass heart and matching fashion sense. Leslie Smith, for the indelible lessons about conscious competence and what it means to fight for your right to pleasure in this world—you're deeply missed, but your legacy lives on inside so many of us. Adaora Asala, for being a ferocious leader on behalf of many communities, and for helping me advise readers on how to refuse to be reduced to symbols. Melissa McEwan, for being an articulate and ornery voice for the voiceless, and for the last-minute save. Deanna Zandt, for her genius solution to the problem of URLs in analog books, and for the long-distance tequila. And Mark Orr, for schooling me about online gaming and virtual worlds, and for the spoons.

Thanks are also owed to the dozens of people who offered up their own personal stories for me to share with you throughout the book. You heard from Ruby Ailment, Chloe Angyal, Cassie Barnes, Elizabeth Calhoun, Jill Filipovic, Idalia Gutierrez, Rachel Casiano Hernández, Miranda Mammen, Laura Mandelberg, Zia Okocha, Simon Pedisich, Renee Randazzo, Jenn Thoman, and Bobbie W., but there were so many more stories I wished I could have shared, from the hilarious to the heartbreaking to the sublime. Thanks to everyone who took the time (and the leap of faith) to send one in.

Obvious but real gratitude is owed to Seal Press, especially Brooke Warner and Merrik Bush-Pirkle, for believing in my vision and helping me make it a reality. Reidan Fredstrom is also owed some applause, for the great good humor to watch me write this entire book on our dining room table and treat it as a fascinating performance-art piece for an audience of one, rather than as the incredible imposition and nuisance I'm sure it was. Thanks to Dave Rini and Andrew Pari for their very necessary last-minute contributions (you know what you did). And, of course, I'm indebted to Colette Perold at *H Bomb,* who first asked the question that inspired this whole project.

Last and most important: I couldn't have even imagined this book without the work of generations of feminist and sex-positive activists, organizers, agitators, evangelists, riot grrrls, zinesters, bloggers, and general troublemakers. I could never finish naming you all, so it hardly seems fair to begin. But know that so much of what I've shared here, I learned from following the trails you blazed. Thank you.

ABOUT THE AUTHOR

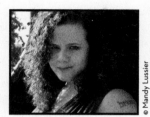

© Mandy Lussier

J ACLYN FRIEDMAN IS A WRITER, PERFORMER, AND ACTIVIST and the editor of the hit book *Yes Means Yes: Visions of Female Sexual Power and a World without Rape* (one of *Publishers Weekly*'s Top 100 Books of 2009).

Friedman is a popular speaker on campuses and at conferences across the United States and beyond. She has been a guest on BBC World Have Your Say, "Democracy Now," *To the Contrary*, and numerous other radio and television shows, and her commentary has appeared in outlets including CNN, *The Washington Post, The Nation*, Jezebel, Feministing.com, *The American Prospect, Bitch*, AlterNet, and *The Huffington Post*. She was named one of 2009's 40 Under 40 by the New Leaders Council.

Friedman is a founder and the executive director of Women, Action & the Media, a national organization working for gender justice in media. She is also a charter member of CounterQuo, a coalition dedicated to challenging the ways we respond to sexual violence.

SELECTED TITLES FROM SEAL PRESS

For more than thirty years, Seal Press has published groundbreaking books. By women. For women.

Yes Means Yes: Visions of Female Sexual Power and A World Without Rape, by Jaclyn Friedman and Jessica Valenti. $16.95, 978-1-58005-257-3. This powerful and revolutionary anthology offers a paradigm shift from the "No Means No" model, challenging men and women to truly value female sexuality and ultimately end rape.

He's A Stud, She's A Slut and 49 Other Double Standards Every Woman Should Know, by Jessica Valenti. $13.95, 978-1-58005-245-0. With sass, humor, and aplomb, Full Frontal Feminism author Jessica Valenti takes on the obnoxious double standards women encounter every day.

The Purity Myth: How America's Obsession with Virginity Is Hurting Young Women, by Jessica Valenti. $16.95, 978-1-58005-314-3. With her usual balance of intelligence and wit, Valenti presents a powerful argument that girls and women, even in this day and age, are overly valued for their sexuality— and that this needs to stop.

F 'em!: Goo Goo, Gaga, and Some Thoughts on Balls, by Jennifer Baumgardner. $17.00, 978-1-58005-360-0. A collection of essays—plus interviews with well-known feminists—by Manifesta co-author Jennifer Baumgardner on everything from purity balls to Lady Gaga.

Outdated: Why Dating Is Ruining Your Love Life, by Samhita Mukhopadhyay. $17.00, 978-1-58005-332-7. An intelligent analysis of how and why young people today are rejecting traditional dating and mating pressures—and why they're better off for doing so.

Kissing Outside the Lines: A True Story of Love and Race and Happily Ever After, by Diane Farr. $24.95, 978-1-58005-390-7. Actress and columnist Diane Farr's unapologetic, and often hilarious, look at the complexities of interracial/ethnic/religious/what-have-you love.

FIND SEAL PRESS ONLINE
www.SealPress.com
www.Facebook.com/SealPress
Twitter: @SealPress